Praise for *Co*

"Campus violence is a complex and multifaceted phenomenon. Campus safety, then, requires a proactive and collaborative approach, supported by effective leadership and on-going commitment. Herein, Hemphill and Hephner LaBanc provide an exceptional framework for addressing campus violence through a range of complementary and collaborative strategies involving public policy, institutional services, and personal commitment. Contributors to this work offer powerful insights regarding strategies to enhance prevention and mitigation of risk, emergency planning and preparation, response to critical incidents, and community recovery. This is a must-read for campus administrators and everyone who is invested in the safety and well-being of our campuses."

— *Gene Deisinger*, Managing Partner, SIGMA Threat Management Associates, P.A.; formerly Deputy Chief of Police and Director, Threat Management Services, Virginia Tech

"NASPA and ACPA remain steadfast in our shared focus to provide practitioners with the knowledge and skills necessary to establish and maintain safe campus environments that are proactive against the threat of devastating violence. Throughout this book, the authors present ideas and practical examples to help campus administrators achieve this end. Because preventing campus homicide and gun violence is an enormous, complex, and critical responsibility placed upon our collective shoulders, sharing knowledge with the higher education community that will build understanding is essential. We hope this resource is helpful as you envision the next steps of your campus's ongoing and evolving effort to prevent and end this violence."

— *Kevin Kruger*, President, NASPA; and *Cindi Love*, Executive Director, ACPA

"*College in the Crosshairs* provides a truly interdisciplinary analysis of phenomena that were once thought of as primarily police responsibilities. As you read this book, prepare to enter the frontline—gun violence, campus safety, and wellness—through the candid voices of the individuals who manage critical operational issues, 24/7, 365. This book is not only edifying for those wishing to learn more about weapons issues but also an indispensable resource for experts in the field. Most of all, this book is deeply inspirational, reminding us that the most powerful weapons against violence are the weapons of peace—education, science, compassion, forgiveness, and courage."

—*Peter F. Lake*, Professor of Law, Charles A. Dana Chair and Director of the Center for Excellence in Higher Education Law and Policy, Stetson University College of Law

COLLEGE IN THE CROSSHAIRS

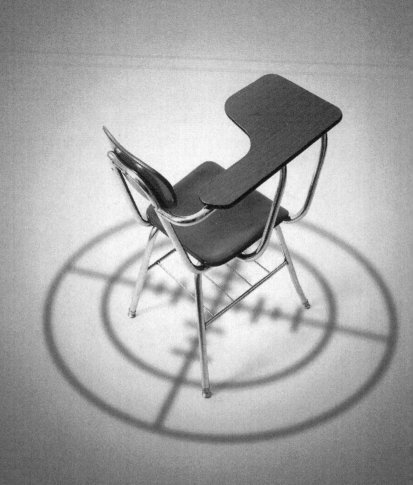

College in the
Crosshairs

An Administrative Perspective on Prevention of Gun Violence

Edited by
Brandi Hephner LaBanc and
Brian O. Hemphill

Foreword by
Kevin Kruger and Cindi Love

A JOINT PUBLICATION OF

STERLING, VIRGINIA

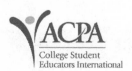

College Student
Educators International

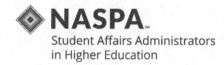

Student Affairs Administrators
in Higher Education

COPYRIGHT © 2015 BY ACPA, COLLEGE
STUDENT EDUCATORS INTERNATIONAL AND
NASPA, THE NATIONAL ASSOCIATION OF
STUDENT PERSONNEL ADMINISTRATORS, INC.

Published by Stylus Publishing, LLC
22883 Quicksilver Drive
Sterling, Virginia 20166-2102

Library of Congress Cataloging-in-Publication-Data
Labanc, Brandi Hephner, 1971-
  College in the crosshairs : an administrative perspective on prevention of gun
violence / edited by Brandi Hephner Labanc and Brian O. Hemphill ; foreword
by Kevin Kruger and Cindi Love.
     pages cm
  Includes index.
  ISBN 978-1-62036-352-2 (pbk. : alk. paper)
  ISBN 978-1-62036-351-5 (cloth : alk. paper)
  ISBN 978-1-62036-353-9 (library networkable e-edition)
  ISBN 978-1-62036-354-6 (consumer e-edition)
  1. Campus violence–United States–Prevention. 2. School shootings–United
States–Prevention. 3. Universities and colleges--Security measures–United
States. 4. Universities and colleges--United States–Safety measures.
  I. Hemphill, Brian O. II. Title.
  LB2866.L32 2015
  371.7'82--dc23
                                            2015012449

  13-digit ISBN: 978-1-62036-351-5 (cloth)
  13-digit ISBN: 978-1-62036-352-2 (paper)
  13-digit ISBN: 978-1-62036-353-9 (library networkable e-edition)
  13-digit ISBN: 978-1-62036-354-6 (consumer e-edition)

Printed in the United States of America

All first editions printed on acid-free paper
that meets the American National Standards Institute
Z39-48 Standard.

Bulk Purchases

Quantity discounts are available for use in workshops
and for staff development.
Call 1-800-232-0223

First Edition, 2015

10   9   8   7   6   5   4   3   2

Contents

3   CREATING AN EMOTIONALLY HEALTHY
COMMUNITY TO PROMOTE CAMPUS SAFETY   76
Maggie Balistreri-Clarke and Peter Meagher

4   STUDENT DEVELOPMENT THEORY IN THE
CAMPUS GUN DEBATE   103
Ainsley Carry and Amy Hecht

5   RISK AND THREAT ASSESSMENT   123
John H. Dunkle and Brian J. Mistler

10 IN HIS WORDS   227
The Tragic Reality
T. Ramon Stuart

11 VIOLENCE PREVENTION IN MODERN ACADEMIA   241
Best Practices for Campus Administrators
Katrina A. Slone and Melanie V. Tucker

ABOUT THE CONTRIBUTORS   271

INDEX   281

Acknowledgments

IT IS WITH GRATEFUL APPRECIATION and sincere indebtedness that we wish to acknowledge the phenomenal work, dedicated focus, and keen attention to detail of Pam Barefield and Katrina A. Slone. We are unendingly appreciative of your support and assistance; truly, this project would not have come to life without your critical involvement, including the countless hours you dedicated to ensuring its success. We would also like to thank our friend Yuma Nakada for again lending his exceptional graphic design talents to this project.

We would like to recognize Daniel W. Jones, chancellor of the University of Mississippi; Morris H. Stocks, provost and vice chancellor for academic affairs at the University of Mississippi; and Tom Susman, chair of the West Virginia State University Board of Governors, whose encouragement and support have allowed us to undertake this expansive and meaningful project.

For their generosity, advocacy, and support, we also wish to acknowledge Kevin Kruger, president of NASPA–Student Affairs Administrators in Higher Education, and Kent Porterfield, past president of ACPA–College Student Educators International, without whom this project could certainly never have come to fruition.

With sincerest gratitude, we would like to express everlasting thankfulness to Dave LaBanc and Marisela Rosas Hemphill, whose staid patience, unending love, and faithful support have provided us an unshakeable foundation. Words simply cannot express our gratitude to each of you for the myriad ways in which you enrich our lives.

Lastly, we would like to remember our dear friend and esteemed colleague Zenobia Lawrence Hikes for the tremendous wisdom and sage counsel she provided during the tragedy we experienced on the

Northern Illinois University campus on February 14, 2008. Though she is no longer with us, her significant work in student affairs set the stage for our country to take action against gun violence in our nation's institutions of higher education in radical new ways. May her legacy continue forever on.

BRIAN O. HEMPHILL
West Virginia State University

BRANDI HEPHNER LABANC
University of Mississippi

Foreword

SHORTLY AFTER MIDNIGHT ON March 18, 2013, students living in the Tower 1 residence hall on the University of Central Florida campus awoke to a fire alarm. Pulling the fire alarm was the first step of a suspect's plan to carry out deadly violence on unsuspecting students living in the hall. Noticing a gun in his possession as students began to evacuate the hall, the suspect's proactive, quick-thinking roommate ran to safety and alerted the police. Within 45 seconds of being notified of a threat, the campus police were on the scene. A quick response prevented another national tragedy and the loss of innocent lives.

The university's review and development of threat assessment and rapid response protocols had begun years prior. And even though the campus's protocol worked, administrators recognized this thwarted tragedy as an opportunity to gather facts and target improvements that could bring about an even more proactive approach to preventing such mass shootings and homicide on campus.

College in the Crosshairs was created out of this recognition—that preventing violence on our campuses is an ongoing, evolving, and necessary leadership responsibility. This is a responsibility in which administrators, particularly those in student affairs, are poised to provide leadership to maintain campus safety. This book also builds on the idea that, by sharing effective practices and resources, we are stronger together.

The authors of the chapters herein provide effective and thoughtful approaches for administrators to design and refine campus policies and procedures to prevent homicidal violence on campus. In chapter 5, for example, authors John H. Dunkle and Brian J. Mistler begin by defining *risk* and *threat assessment* and build upon this definition by describing various frameworks that campus leaders can use to create and establish a campuswide risk assessment team.

Effective teams, these authors point out, cultivate a communitywide approach to campus safety by empowering members to report suspicious behavior.

A critical component of establishing a communitywide approach to preventing campus shootings and murders is integrating technology as a resource to both report threats and notify the community of potential or imminent danger. Though technology is highly useful, the integration of this resource into campus violence prevention efforts is one to approach with careful consideration. In chapter 7, Jeanna Mastrodicasa and Greg Nayor outline best practices and strategies for providing timely notification, particularly in times of crisis, to the campus community.

As we examine our campuses' approaches to such violence prevention, it is important to recognize, too, that what works best may differ between campuses. This is especially true when our duty to maintain campus safety is met with the constant challenges of strained resources and limited staff. Framing two case examples and identifying a set of best practices, Steve Jacobson and Sheila Lambert provide campus administrators with a detailed view of what preventing shootings and killings looks like at small colleges in chapter 8.

Though we work diligently to prevent campus homicide, we do not always know if and when this violence will strike our communities. In chapter 1, Rick Ferraro shares the sobering reality that, in the years following the Virginia Tech tragedy and despite heavy efforts nationwide to stop university-connected homicides, the incidence of such violence has not declined. This affirms the critical importance of remaining vigilant and continuing to build upon our prevention efforts. In chapter 11, Katrina A. Slone and Melanie V. Tucker delve into best practices to continuously and carefully implement strategies that reduce the likelihood of mass shootings and similar violence. Ongoing efforts to reduce the threat are both imperative and personal to professionals like Lance Jones, who, through his account in chapter 9 with Scott Peska of responding to an active shooter emergency at Casper College, helps us to understand and build upon our prevention and rapid response strategies, particularly in the community college setting.

The thought and intentionality we put toward the technical aspects of how we design and administer our approaches to preventing shootings and murders are, of course, essential to affirming our duty of care to students. But how we nurture our community members, particularly students who navigate the personal and societal difficulties associated with mental illness, is also central to affirming a safe environment. As we continue to reexamine the approaches we take to ensure campus safety, it is imperative for us to carefully consider whether our students are provided with the level of support they need. And in the context of campus safety, this is a compelling example of the value we as student affairs professionals bring to students we serve. We demonstrate value through the capacity to establish clear and effective administrative practices to achieve campus safety while integrating an educational and developmental focus with students.

Being educationally and developmentally focused within the campus safety task means addressing—within ourselves and elsewhere on the campus—the stigmas and stereotypes associated with mental illness. We should establish practices that nurture those who need help, including students who have been identified as posing a potential threat to campus safety. Moreover, we can educate our community about what a healthy campus environment looks like, challenging ignorance and affirming acceptance and inclusion. These ideas are elevated by Maggie Balistreri-Clarke and Peter Meagher in chapter 3, in which the authors discuss practices and strategies to build a sense of ownership and an emotionally healthy community in the context of campus safety and violence prevention.

But how should we affirm students who may pose a potential threat to the safety of themselves and others as members of our campus community? Absent a reason to believe a threat is present, one common approach is to monitor these students as they interact with fellow members of the campus community. In chapter 6, Jen Day Shaw and Sarah B. Westfall build on this practice by encouraging professionals to complement monitoring with interventions that support and nurture these students according to their individual needs. The authors describe how we can assess our students of concern and, in turn, establish a set of accommodations and services to nurture these individuals as members of the campus community.

Building and affirming a sense of community are also essential to how a campus and its students process and manage grief and reconciliation after a traumatic event. This was the goal of T. Ramon Stuart, who, in chapter 10, describes how students were brought together to process the emotions associated with the death of one student and the homicide of another. And at the heart of processing these emotions is an opportunity to connect how we support the emotional health of our students with student development theory.

In the years after the tragedy at Virginia Tech, public concern about campus shootings and other deadly violence has risen to a crescendo. From the White House to state legislatures across the country, the appropriate public policy response to deal with the threat of violence has been a persistent and commanding source of debate. And the debate has been intense and deeply divided, with some advocates calling for stricter gun regulations whereas others are pushing to allow individuals to carry firearms on campus if they so choose. As policy makers consider the place of firearms on our campuses, Ainsley Carry and Amy Hecht frame Kohlberg's moral development theory in the context of the debate through an engaging discussion in chapter 4, encouraging us to ask whether our students are developmentally ready to make a morally sophisticated, life-changing decision to use firearms in response to a real or perceived threat. These and similar considerations signal that, as Kerry Brian Melear and Mark St. Louis eloquently posit in chapter 2, "higher education stands at a point of transition . . . and has certainly earned the right to participate as a salient voice in the public policy debate to help shape the contours of gun control legislation in the United States."

Because we hold a duty of care to our students and are responsible for the safety of our campuses, we should act as agents of responsible policy by adding to the conversation with lawmakers, campus leaders, and the public about what it takes to keep our communities safe. But we should also act as responsible stewards of our campuses, acting in good faith to comply with the legal and regulatory framework in which we practice. To this end, Melear and St. Louis offer examples of recent legal decisions that help us to be informed and current in our roles.

As the leading associations for the study and practice of the student affairs profession, NASPA–Student Affairs Administrators in Higher Education and ACPA–College Student Educators International seek to provide resources that will enable administrators to leverage effective practices where they exist and target areas worth our attention. It is our hope that this book offers perspectives and approaches that allow you to elevate new ideas and approaches that strengthen violence prevention protocols on your campus and affirm a nurturing educational community for students.

NASPA and ACPA remain steadfast in our shared focus to provide practitioners with the knowledge and skills necessary to establish and maintain safe campus environments that are proactive against the threat of devastating violence. Throughout this book, the authors present ideas and practical examples to help campus administrators achieve this end. Because preventing campus homicide and gun violence is an enormous, complex, and critical responsibility placed upon our collective shoulders, sharing knowledge with the higher education community that will build upon our knowledge and understanding is essential. We hope this resource is helpful as you envision the next steps of your campus's ongoing and evolving effort to prevent and end this violence.

KEVIN KRUGER, PHD
President, NASPA–Student Affairs Administrators in Higher Education

CINDI LOVE, EDD
Executive Director, ACPA–College Student Educators International

1 Murder in Academe

An Overview of Rampage Shootings and More Conventional Homicides That Touch Universities and Colleges (2009–2014)

Rick Ferraro

THIS CHAPTER, divided into three parts, gives an overview of homicides that have touched public and private universities and colleges in the United States from January 2009 through June 2014. The first part of this chapter deals with that most extraordinary phenomenon, "rampage shooting events"; then, conventional homicides on college campuses are explored. Finally, reforms and recommendations are offered in the third section.

Rampage shootings have no exact definition, and there is no precise set of elements that applies to all cases, yet these shootings frequently share characteristics from among the following:

> ➤ Casualties (killed and injured) tend to be higher than with common crimes (e.g., burglary or mugging). Some researchers may use a minimal statistical guideline of four victims to help define *rampage shootings*.[1]
> ➤ The cause often is unclear, exaggerated, or incomprehensible. For example, delusional notions, rather than concrete grievances or objectives, may serve as cause to act.
> ➤ The target(s) can be varied and arbitrary. A large, ill-defined group based on ready access rather than a specific person(s) may be targeted.
> ➤ The shooting event can involve multiple and/or complex target sites.[2]
> ➤ The event can be driven by grandiose thinking. Rampage killing is often seen by the shooter as an event of long-term historical

1

significance that will retroactively redeem and justify a life that, to the wider world, would seem a fundamental failure.[3]

These five dynamic elements—casualty rate, unclear motives, variable targets, multisiting, and grandiose thinking—increase the potential for an oversized impact on the physical, mental, social, and economic well-being of a community.

The second part of this chapter deals with semiextraordinary or more conventional murder, which tends to focus on actions taken against one or two individuals. Still, one should not underestimate the negative impact that conventional murder can have on a campus. When we deal with a capital domestic incident, a fatal sexual assault, or a bruising death from hazing, the impact, qualitatively, can be profound.[4]

The linking of the two parts—rampage and conventional violence— is deliberate. Homicide exists on a continuum. By understanding better the entire picture as it relates to the willful taking of life, both on the grand and lesser scales, we can do more to try to prevent the same. Safety and security measures and programming in the interest of promoting prosocial behavior can be applied across the board.

Finally, there is no purpose in wading through so many stories of inhumanity and heartache unless it is to learn from these experiences and to help bring about reform. The third part of this chapter looks to that hopeful end.

Rampage Shooters and Their Violence

On April 16, 2007, Seung-Hui Cho, a 23-year-old undergraduate, slew 32 members of the Virginia Tech (VT) community, injured 27 others, and then took his own life. High casualties and a high killed-to-wounded ratio occurred for two reasons: (a) Cho secured the entering doors to Norris Hall with heavy chains and delayed the relieving column of police for several critical minutes; and (b) Cho repeatedly fired into the bodies of the fallen.[5]

In the immediate aftermath, professional and amateur journalists, in traditional mass media and in the blogosphere, suggested a plethora of "interesting" explanations for the event:

1. *Political*: Cho was a follower of Al-Qaeda or suffered from post-traumatic stress disorder (PTSD) due to military service (Lee, 2007).

2. *Familial*: His parents were abusive, remote, or unsupportive.[6]
3. *Pedagogical*: His teachers were overly lenient or too demanding.[7]
4. *Religious*: His Muslim or Catholic views, or demonic possession, were to blame (Adams, 2007).[8]
5. *Medicinal*: Alcohol, illegal drugs, antidepressants, or antianxiety medications were at fault (Williams, 2007).
6. *Discrimination*: He suffered from anti-Asian or anti-immigrant bigotry.[9]
7. *Bullying*: The shooter had been bullied at VT.[10]

In fact, Cho was an apolitical civilian; his family was supportive; teachers worked with him in a fair manner; he was not religious; he did not consume alcohol or take legal or illegal drugs; he was not subject to discrimination at VT; and far from bullying him, students, faculty, and staff at VT tried to befriend him.

Shortly after the tragedy, students set out a 33rd "Hokie Stone," or limestone marker, for Cho. Placed on the historic drill field, next to those for the 32 fallen innocents, the memorial conveyed the charitable assumption that Cho was not responsible for his acts due to mental illness. The gesture underlined that, despite his grievous offenses, the bell metaphorically would still toll for him (Associated Press, 2007).

The 33rd stone was permanently removed by students only after Cho's video diatribe (sent to NBC News) went viral. Therein, Cho declared his acts to be knowing and intentional; he spewed hateful words to all; and with perfect vainglory, he lavished praise and pity upon himself.

Cho, while alive, obscured his spirit and countenance through extreme reticence, dark glasses, and pulled-down caps. In death, by bitter actions and words, he made himself an island—isolated and unconnected from those with whom he should have shared fellowship in life and memory. To this day his name is almost never uttered on campus; if allusion is made to him it is in the abstract—to "the shooter."

For some months after "4/16," I took solace in the fact that Cho seemed to represent something *sui generis* and that his actions were a stand-alone event in the context of higher education. He appeared to personify the brutal rampage killer, who had been encountered only very rarely. In 2007, to find a roughly comparable event, I had to go back over 40 years to the Bell Tower shootings at the University of Texas at Austin in 1966 (Lavergne, 1997).

However, less than a year later, on February 14, 2008, Steven Kazmierczak, a recent 27-year-old graduate from Northern Illinois University (NIU), at the time enrolled in graduate study at the University of Illinois, returned to his alma mater. Entering an auditorium-style classroom of perhaps 120 souls, Kazmierczak opened fire with a shotgun and a handgun, hitting 25 people and killing 5, before he finally dispatched himself (Vann, 2009).

It was also disturbing to find a conscious link among rampage shooters. Klebold and Harris of Columbine had inspired Cho, who in turn served as a warped role model for Kazmierczak. As I finished writing an essay entitled "Violence in the Shadow of the Ivory Tower," in 2009, with the collaboration of Blanche McHugh, I wondered what the future would hold. Would rampage killing in higher education become commonplace? Were Cho and Kazmierczak not isolated islands but rather bodies in a dark archipelago which would emerge as if from a fog, endangering collegiate wayfarers on their journey?

Therefore, we ask where we have gone after the signal events of 2007 and 2008 at VT and NIU. In the time that has passed from January 2009 through June 2014, have things gotten better? Are they worse? Or do they look roughly the same?

Assessing University or College Rampage Shooters: A Census for January 2009–June 2014

The archetypal university or college rampage shooter seems to embody the following five constituent elements:

1. The shooter is a current or recent university/college affiliate.
2. The shooter uses a handgun and/or rifle.
3. The shooter kills a significant number of people—say, not less than three or four.
4. The attack takes place at the university/college.
5. There is no legal justification for the event—for example, the shooter is not acting in self-defense.

So, let us map and score the candidates and events that took place over nearly six years against the criteria.

1. **December 8, 2009, Jason Hamilton at Northern Virginia Community College.** On December 8, 2009, 20-year-old Hamilton entered a campus math class in which he had earned a failing grade, drew a hunting rifle out of a hockey bag, and fired twice at his math teacher. Hamilton missed, in part because his aim was high and in part because his female instructor ducked. He tried to shoot a third time, but his rifle jammed. He then walked into an adjacent hallway to await arrest. In March 2011, Hamilton pleaded guilty to attempted murder (Barakat, 2011).

   ➤ Score: 4 of 5 elements. Hamilton caused psychological distress for his teacher and other students, but due to misaim and misfire, he killed or wounded no one.

2. **February 12, 2010, Professor Amy Bishop at the University of Alabama in Huntsville.** A current professor using a 9-mm handgun, Bishop killed three colleagues and wounded three more in a departmental meeting on campus. Disappointment at not being tenured did not justify murder (Keefe, 2013).

   ➤ Score: 5 of 5.

3. **September 28, 2010, Colton Tooley at the University of Texas at Austin.** Tooley, a 19-year-old sophomore, dressed in a dark suit and ski mask, and carrying an AK-47 assault rifle, fired 11 times in the air on campus grounds before moving into the Perry-Castenada Library, where he fatally shot himself on the sixth floor near the children's book section (Daily Mail Reporter, 2010). Some see this as a purely suicidal event, with dark suit, mask, and public firing as stagecraft (Woods, 2010). Others wonder if it was a political statement: Tooley came from a house divided on gun control, and a campus speaker was set to talk about the issue shortly. Yet there is no known justification for his having carried and fired a semiautomatic assault rifle (Finnegan, 2010).

   ➤ Score: 4 of 5. Tooley caused distress for others as gunshot sounds were compounded by institutional memory (this was the same campus in which Charles Whitman conducted a rampage event in 1966); however, Tooley killed only one person—himself.

4. **January 8, 2011, Jared Lee Loughner at a Safeway shopping center in Arizona.** Congresswoman Gabrielle Giffords was hosting a reception for constituents at a shopping center in Tucson, Arizona, when Loughner, a recent student at Pima Community College, opened fire with a 9-mm Glock fed by a 30-bullet clip, killing 6 people and wounding 14 others, including Giffords ("Collection," n.d.). The shooting ceased when he was brought down by bystanders as he tried to pick up a dropped ammunition clip (Kennedy, 2011). Loughner had been suspended (not permanently dismissed) from Pima Community College in October 2010, due to disruptive, harassing, and threatening behavior ("Jared Loughner Had," 2011).

   ➢ Score: 4 of 5. The shooting occurred off campus, yet featured a strong school link because Loughner (wrongly) placed blame on the college. His parents also saw the suspension as "putting him over the edge." Pima officials actually had recommended that Loughner seek treatment in time away from study, but this recommendation was not followed. The suspension, instead of being a time to repair and retool, became the excuse for an explosion of violence off campus.

5. **December 11, 2011, Ross Ashley on the campus of VT.** Ashley, a 22-year-old student at Radford University, drove to nearby VT and fatally shot VT police officer Deriek Crouse as he was issuing a ticket to a person who had no connection with either Crouse or Ashley. Also, Crouse and Ashley shared no personal or legal history. Two possibilities come to mind: (a) Ashley committed a thrill kill; or (b) this shooting was part of a larger, rampage plan. If it were the latter, the speed with which police responded may have spurred Ashley's decision to commit suicide and prevented additional casualties (Lewis & Sampson, 2011).

> Score: 4 of 5. Ashley was a shooter, employed a gun, and acted without justification. He is counted as a current student because he was enrolled at Radford. He may have come to VT to act out the tragedy on a larger stage. The short casualty list (two dead) does not fit the classic picture of a rampage event.

6. **April 2, 2012, One L. Goh at Oikos University.** A 43-year-old student, upset by tuition charges, and carrying a handgun with extended ammunition clips, Goh killed 7 people and wounded 3 others, firing in a classroom and a university parking lot (Kang, 2013).

   > Score: 5 of 5. Goh, a naturalized citizen, complained that people made fun of his accented English, but that did not justify mass murder (Collins, 2012).

7. **July 20, 2012, James Holmes at the Century 16 (now Century Aurora) movie theater.** Holmes was a graduate student who had dropped out of his doctoral program at the University of Colorado Medical Center in Aurora due to academic difficulty. Armed with a shotgun, a rifle, handguns, thousands of rounds of ammunition, a knife, and tear gas canisters, he killed 12 people and wounded 58 others in an Aurora movie theater (Lutz, 2012).

   > Score: 4 of 5. The theater was an off-campus establishment. However, the account closely involved the school because Holmes was contemplating homicide while enrolled (as we know from a counselor's timely warning to police). In addition, it is likely that this attack was a misplaced response to academic disappointment.

8. **December 14, 2012, Adam Lanza at Sandy Hook Elementary School.** In an attack that began at home, 20-year-old Lanza killed his mother, a gun enthusiast, who took her son to shooting ranges and who had gifted him weapons (Flegenheimer, 2013). Lanza then drove to Sandy Hook Elementary School, which he had attended as a child. Having taken a rifle and handgun from a veritable arsenal at home, he killed 26 people, including 6 adults and 20 small

children, in fewer than 5 minutes.[11] Then, with police approaching, he shot himself. Lanza had been enrolled at Western Connecticut State University in 2008–2009, as a joint-enrollment student (Associated Press, 2012).[12]

> ➤ Score: 3 of 5. Lanza is mainly viewed as a secondary school student put in a university dual program because he could not operate socially in high school. Although there is no direct connection to a university, Lanza was affected by college and university rampage killing and was fascinated by the mass shooting that took place at NIU in 2008. A second point can be deducted because Sandy Hook did not have even a tangential connection with a university or collegiate program.

9. **March 18, 2013, James Seevakumaran at the University of Central Florida.** Seevakumaran, a 30-year-old student, spoke negatively about his mixed-race heritage and directed racist expressions toward others ("James Seevakumaran," 2013). He planned to kill as many people as possible in his residence hall of 500, and, to that end, had acquired a rifle, a handgun, thousands of rounds of ammunition, and 4 Molotov cocktails. He would pull a fire alarm to get everyone into the open, and then he would fire. But his roommate, trying to check for smoke related to the alarm, encountered Seevakumaran with what he thought was an assault rifle in hand (it was actually a semiautomatic .22-caliber rifle) and ran and locked himself into a bathroom ("UCF Gunman," 2013). There the roommate dialed 911. With police on the way, Seevakumaran shot himself fatally with the handgun.

> ➤ Score: 4 of 5. Seevakumaran was the only casualty.

10. **April 10, 2013, Dylan Andrew Quick at Lone Star College, CyFair Campus.** Quick, who was born deaf, claimed—after he had been arrested—that he had been bullied (Nelson, 2013). However, by virtue of a cochlear implant, and his constant attendance at a reading club associated with the campus library, Quick quickly made up ground, and came to be admired

as an academic and personal role model by library staff. That was before April 2013, when this 20-year-old student went on a building-to-building rampage on campus, in which he stabbed 14 students with a scalpel or X-Acto knife. Hospitals reported 2 students in critical condition and 6 others in fair condition as a result (Plushnick-Masti & Lozano, 2013).

➤ Score: 4 of 5. Quick killed no one, but the injury count was high, and wounds were serious.

11. **April 12, 2013, Neil Allen MacInnis at New River Community College in Virginia.** MacInnis, age 18, a student of New River Community College, entered a satellite facility of the college, located at a shopping mall (Associated Press, 2013). MacInnis, who had previously attended a police academy program for citizens, had posted his planned attack online shortly before he opened fire with a legally purchased shotgun (Shaw, 2013). He hit two females, a fellow student, and a part-time employee, whom he did not know (Powell, 2014). He also called out, pretending to be a police officer, so people might emerge from hiding, and he had thought about pulling a fire alarm so as to assemble a larger target (Powell, 2014). He was apprehended in the parking lot by an unarmed off-duty security guard who told him to put down his rifle, which he did (Atkins, 2013). Having pled guilty to four felony charges in April 2014, he faces 38 years in prison.

➤ Score: 4 of 5. MacInnis fit all the categories save for the high casualty rate. He injured two people seriously, but not critically, and he surrendered when told to do so. However, MacInnis was not expert in the use of guns (as he himself shared in a video), so the nonfatal outcome may be partially attributed to relative incompetence.

12. **June, 2013, John Zawahri, including Santa Monica College.** Zawahri, age 23, was a recent student at Santa Monica City College, where his father and brother also attended. In June 2013, he engaged in a shooting spree that commenced with the gunning down of his father and brother at the family

house, which he set on fire (Brown, 2013). Then the conflict spilled out onto the streets, where he hijacked a car and fired shots at buses and automobiles. It ended in the library of Santa Monica City College. He killed 5 people, wounded 4 others, and was finally shot mortally by police. Wearing a tactical vest, he used a semiautomatic rifle; wore a .44-caliber revolver; and had extended magazines with 30 bullets each. He also carried a duffel bag stuffed with ammunition (Abcarian, Garrison, & Groves, 2013).

➢ Score: 5 of 5.

13. **May 23, 2014, Elliot Rodger and the Santa Barbara murders.**[13] Rodger, age 22, had an urbane style in his writing and was soft-spoken in his YouTube videos. Yet, he was seething with frustration and hate; he talked of wanting to kill all women and all sexually active men. Moreover, he was merciless in his actions, using a knife and a hammer, several guns, and his BMW automobile over multiple sites (his apartment, the grounds of a sorority house, and the streets of Santa Barbara) to kill 6 people and wound 13 others before killing himself.

➢ Score: 5 of 5.

14. **June 5, 2014, Aaron Ybarra at Seattle Pacific University.** Twenty-six-year-old Ybarra killed one student, seriously injured a second, and caused a third to be hit by shrapnel at Seattle Pacific University (Jonsson, 2014). Ybarra had been on this campus only once before, when he pretended to be a candidate for admission (to scout it as a shooting sight). He brought a shotgun and 50 shells and had 25 more shells in his truck. He also had some experience with guns because he had worked at a shooting range.

➢ Score: 5 of 5. Ybarra was a recent student; though he never enrolled at Seattle Pacific, he attended Edmonds Community College sporadically from 2005 to 2012.

Overall Assessment

In reply to the query, "Have things gotten better, worse, or stayed about the same?": From 2009 to 2014, with respect to the frequency of rampage events that have a university/collegiate connection, in truth, matters have gotten worse. There are 14 events and 14 people, a great deal of activity in a short time span.

Five events featured all five elements associated with a classic university/college rampage shooting. Eight others were strongly related to four constituent elements. Only one (the Sandy Hook massacre) represents a bit of a stretch, though events related to university/collegiate life exercised some influence.

In terms of intensity, the events, both singly and grouped, were tragic: Oikos University suffered 10 students killed or wounded, a significant portion of the population at a small school (Wood, 2012); the University of California, Santa Barbara lost 6 students ("In Memory," 2014); the University of Alabama in Huntsville had an important academic department decimated (Wadman, 2010); Sandy Hook lost 26 people, many veritable babies; Aurora, Colorado, saw 70 people killed or injured at a movie house; and Tucson, Arizona, suffered great losses from Loughner, a man who had always insisted on his "free speech rights," as he harassed others at school and not only shot many but also almost silenced the free speech of a U.S. congresswoman.[14] Multisited shootings—as at Santa Monica and Santa Barbara—shattered the notion of a secure border between on campus and off campus. Instead, the shootings underlined that gun violence is extremely permeable, and shooters do not have to await an entry permit to cross in either direction.

Do the events with fewer fatalities say something positive? It may be that people like Tooley and MacInnis failed to kill others because some part of their conscience took over at the last moment; less optimistically, they may simply have lost their nerve, or they may have been too psychically disorganized to do what they truly wanted. We should also keep in mind that in at least five cases, jammed guns limited the havoc. In another case, the selected weapon—a knife—turned out to be very good for cruel wounding but not for thorough killing, making the low fatality rate a function of the chosen equipment.

The one optimistic point to underline is the heroic action of some bystanders. In four of the cases, rampage killers were stopped or slowed down by people working together. In two instances, people used their collective muscle; in another, a nonfatal spray of Mace did the trick; and in yet another case, it was an authoritative command from an unarmed security guard—people all working without guns. In the Tucson incident, however, there was almost an unintentional tragedy. A well-meaning passerby, carrying his own handgun, almost shot another man who had just wrestled a gun away from Jared Loughner. Happily, the potential for friendly fire was avoided by the timely cries of helpful, unarmed bystanders on the scene (Saletan, 2011).

Some Demographic Characteristics of This Group of Shooters

There are myriad opinions about the reasons shooters do what they do—gender, access to guns, mental illness, societal failings, and so on. So what commonalities exist? Are there demographic themes related to these rampage shootings? The review of each case provides clarity related to these characteristics and themes.

Type of School, Gender, Ethnicity, Age, and Level

Perhaps with incidents at the University of Texas, VT, and NIU in mind, I had expected that community colleges would really not be much mentioned with respect to rampage shooters. However, half of the 14 incidents related to higher education in the timeframe examined in this study were drawn from community college ranks.

Of the 14 rampage killers for the period under review, 13 were males. This is not particularly surprising, because for biological and sociological reasons violence has more commonly been associated with men. However, the mentalities of these 13 males and the depths to which they fell are extraordinary. They engaged in violence with no purpose. Absent were not only modern notions of masculinity but also classic notions of a man as "protector of the weak," bulwark for family, or provider of justice.

Turning to women, in my 2008 research stretching back to 1965, I could locate only one female rampage killer who touched on academe. Jillian Robbins, a 19-year-old army reservist, as part of a murder/suicide plan, sniped at Penn State students on campus in 1996. She killed one female student; seriously wounded a male international student; barely missed two other students (bullets went through their backpacks); and attempted to stab a fifth student, who disarmed her. But Robbins was never a college student at Penn State or anywhere else (Gibb, 2003). The first female member of a university community to qualify as a rampage killer is the aforementioned professor, Amy Bishop, who shot six colleagues and would have hit more if her gun had not jammed.

Many people assume that rampage shooters are disproportionately White. However, it might be fairer to say that this list resembles America. Among the White group are people from English, Greek, Irish, Italian, and Scottish backgrounds. Asia, Korea, Lebanon, Malaysia, and India are represented, and we list one person of Hispanic origin and another likely of mixed Hispanic origin. The only numerically significant group missing is African Americans, which seemingly flies in the face of prevailing social stereotypes that blame Black youth for violence in America.

With respect to age, 2 of the people listed were in their early 40s. Four others were between 25 and 31, and 8 were between 18 and 23. Therefore, concerns are seen in traditional and nontraditional age groups.

In terms of educational status, one offender was a professor, one was a graduate student, one was a dual enrollment student, and 10 were undergraduates. Eight attacked their own school, four attacked another school, two attacked outside targets, and two attacked more than one site. Finally, all the attackers had a background in academe, and some held scholarships. Instead of being grateful for a college education, however, they turned on their alma maters.

Psychological and Emotional Issues

In reading about most of these figures, I feel like I should have Virgil as a guide, for we seem to be entering Dante's *Purgatorio*. The actions are so dark that in many ways the subject matter feels more like an exploration of deadly sins than the unfolding of psychological conditions with fatal consequences. Perhaps if one is too many standard deviations away from basic goodness, one arrives at the intersection of moral uncleanliness and insanity. Or it could be that when the wrath of a rampage killer is unleashed, we approach the term *madness* both psychologically and emotionally. Putting these speculations aside, let us summarize on a case-by-case basis what we know as seen through the lens of abnormal psychology and mental illness.

1. *Jason Hamilton*: At his plea hearing, his lawyer stated that Hamilton had serious mental health issues but would not be specific. A court-ordered evaluation agreed but also found that Hamilton was still legally responsible. At that proceeding, he faced 2–20 years in prison, with the mental health issues perhaps making the difference between a shorter or longer sentence ("Jason Hamilton," 2011).

2. *Amy Bishop*: Her lawyer openly suggested that she was paranoid schizophrenic, but then he retreated, saying that that might not be the case (James, 2010). There was initial talk of an insanity defense. However, Bishop eventually took a plea that made no mention of mental illness, but removed the death penalty and effectively assigned her life in prison without parole (Associated Press, 2012).

3. *Colton Tooley*: Tooley described himself as "socially detached"; others said he was intelligent, reserved, and incapable of hurting a fly. His relatives did not believe that he was depressed. However, Tooley did commit suicide (Shannon, 2010).

4. *Jared Loughner*: He consumed alcohol and drugs (marijuana and hallucinogens) heavily (Cloud, 2011). In legal proceedings, court-appointed experts estimated that he was paranoid schizophrenic (Lacey, 2011). Further, although the Court of Appeals at first ruled that Loughner could not be compelled to take antipsychotic medication, the panel shortly thereafter reversed its decision because his behavior was deteriorating drastically, and he was becoming highly suicidal. Once those medications were taken, his behavior improved significantly ("Jared Loughner to Be Forced," 2011). Loughner was sentenced to life in prison.

5. *Ross Ashley*: Ashley had broken up with a girlfriend during the previous summer but did not seem very upset. Friends mentioned family friction, but it seemed within normal bounds. A number of

people pointed to small matters, including cursing loudly on the phone, running up and down the apartment corridor, and going to the same shooting range used by Seung-Hui Cho. But these may indicate nothing beyond slight eccentricity or coincidence. His parents released a short statement expressing regret for the event but indicated that they would have no further comment. Official sources cited HIPAA, which suggests that Ashley might have had at least some contact with a counselor at school or elsewhere, but no specific information has been forthcoming. Ashley committed suicide (Caulfield, 2011).

6. *One L. Goh*: In court proceedings, two court-appointed forensic psychologists found that Goh was paranoid schizophrenic (Associated Press, 2013). Goh has been confined to a mental hospital and is still not ready to stand trial. If judged competent to be tried, he could face the death penalty. Also, schizophrenia was found in his family's history, with two close relatives having been affected (Kang, 2013).

7. *James Holmes*: Holmes had talked with more than one psychological therapist associated with the University of Colorado–Denver campus (Coffman, 2012). He also sent a message to another graduate student and inquired about "dysphoric mania"—a condition that can lead to paranoid delusions—warning that person to stay away from him "because [he] was bad news" (McLaughlin, 2012). He had been prescribed antidepressant and antianxiety medications; he also mentioned to a stranger that he took LSD and other hallucinogens (Ferner, 2013). Holmes also played a lot of violent video games. He talked about suicidal/homicidal ideation, which university psychiatrist Lynne Fenton shared appropriately to give timely warning to campus police (Ingold, 2013). It is said that Holmes made threats against a professor and was barred from campus, but the university denied that assertion. In a filing by prosecutors, Holmes reputedly said that he wanted to kill people when his life was over. Holmes's defense team, early in proceedings, offered to take an "insanity plea" if that would remove the death penalty option. Holmes was found guilty on 24 counts of first-degree murder, 140 counts of attempted first-degree murder, 1 count of possessing explosives, and a sentence enhancement of a crime of violence. He was sentenced to life in

prison without the possibility of parole. Holmes sent a packet to Dr. Fenton just before his rampage, which likely talks about his intentions and state of mind; if the contents are ever shared publicly, they may be enlightening. In addition, an encrypted mental health report on Holmes was completed by therapists at the Colorado Mental Health Institute in Pueblo. It was sent to the court, but it has been legally sealed (Ferner, 2013).

8. *Adam Lanza*: Initially Lanza was said to have "sensory disintegration disorder," which sounds arguably more descriptive than clinical ("Report Says," 2013). Others pointed to Asperger's syndrome, obsessive-compulsive disorder, and depression (Nano, 2012). His father believes he was schizophrenic and that the Asperger's obscured that fact (Nye, 2014). When he was 11 or 12, Lanza resisted antidepressant medication prescribed by therapists at the Yale Child Study Center, ostensibly due to side effects; his mother supported that resistance (Griffin, 2013). More ominously, both mother and son may have been resistant to treatment, hoping to work out problems through accommodations and extra attention rather than through addressing core issues. In addition, Lanza may have had pedophiliac tendencies—his computer contains a play that centers on the sexual relationship of a 30-year-old man and 10-year-old child—which may help explain his target of a primary school (Chapman, 2014). He was exposed to vicarious violence to an extraordinary degree and may have been highly desensitized; one source says he racked up 83,000 kills online, including 22,000 head shots; and in his room there were pictures of mutilated corpses, including those of children (Lysiak, 2013). Moreover, he was obsessed with people who had engaged in mass shootings (Fox, 2013). Lanza also had a body mass index (BMI) of 15.2, consistent with disordered eating. Finally, Lanza committed not only matricide and a version of infanticide but also suicide.

9. *James Seevakumaran*: Seevakumaran never sought counseling at the University of Central Florida (Colby, Hamacher, & Finch, 2013). He had an alter ego named Damien, featured in a short, crude three-page letter. Damien, a mixed-race man, hated African Americans, referring to them with the "N-word"; he referred to White people using the "H-word" (Sadowsky, 2013). Damien's

plan for revenge was the same one that Seevakumaran would put into play: Pull the fire alarm, fire on the assembled masses, and then commit suicide. In a second note found in Seevakumaran's room, there was the exhortation, "Hate is the key." It sounds like the student was trying to work himself up into a fury.

10. *Dylan Quick*: After he was apprehended, Quick volunteered to police authorities some aspects of his life, including the following: He had fantasies about people that involved stabbing, skinning, cannibalism, and necrophilia, fantasies that went back to his eighth birthday. In his apartment, police found a latex Hannibal Lector mask (Lozano, 2013).

11. *Neil MacInnis*: MacInnis's relatives said they knew of no reason why MacInnis would become violent. However, he had written a story in high school on a school shooter, and a cell phone video that he produced prior to the shooting suggested mental illness. Further, in other videos that MacInnis made, he compared himself with the shooters of VT, Columbine, and Aurora (Starviego, 2013). In high school MacInnis had thought about bringing a gun to class to engage in a rampage event, but he was too young to buy one (Powell, 2014). Despite mentioning what seems to be a dissociative state (blacked out), he makes a sane and logical recommendation: "We need to have something where people can't hurt people. . . . It's just real easy to get guns." (Powell, 2014). In regard to suicide, MacInnis acknowledges in one of his videos that he was feeling somewhat suicidal and that he had attempted to kill himself in 2010, but he also noted that if the rampage went well, he might not have to take his own life (Powell, 2014). Finally, courts did determine that MacInnis was mentally competent and could stand trial.

12. *John Zawahri*: In high school, Zawahri had been admitted to the University of California, Los Angeles's Neuropsychiatric Institute for assessment and treatment. While attending alternative high school in 2006, he had been observed searching the Internet in order to learn how to make explosives, resulting in psychiatric referral. When police conducted a search at his home, they found bomb-making materials. He also made threats against students and teachers in high school (Abcarian, Garrison, & Groves, 2013).

13. *Elliot Rodger*: Rodger had consistent access to expert psychological care, and he had strong support from his parents and stepparents. At various points, his issues were attributed to autism generally, Asperger's syndrome, and/or depression. His lengthy autobiography, "My Twisted Life," contains a lot of misogynistic content (e.g., he proposes prison camps for women), but he also showed a visceral dislike for most men (and he actually killed more men than women). In addition, Rodger was uneasy with his biracial heritage, and directed racist comments toward African Americans, Hispanics, and Asians. He exhibited class prejudice and was obsessed with material wealth. However, his core issue—the one that produced the greatest rage and the most frequent episodes of self-pity—was his virginal status. In his mind, there was only one way in which the drought of forced celibacy could be relieved; at least one tall, beautiful, blonde woman had to throw herself at Rodger and take his virginity. (It was rather like the sleeping beauty waiting for the prince's kiss, but in reverse.) Rodger was quite clear that his celibacy issue could not be resolved by engaging a paid escort, having sex with an uncomely woman, or even fostering initial interest by paying a compliment to an attractive woman. Narcissism and vanity, of unaccustomed intensity, in the end, seem to have been the most destructive forces in his life (Rodger, 2014b).

14. *Aaron Ybarra*: Ybarra had stopped taking psychotropic medication because "he wanted to feel hate" (Associated Press, 2014). On the day of the shooting at Seattle Pacific, he wrote that he wanted people to die; he volunteered that he wanted to die, as well. He was drawn to Columbine, indicating that he had heard the voice of Eric Harris, the more pathological of the two Colorado killers (Jonsson, 2014). In addition, Ybarra expressed admiration for the shooter at VT. His psychological background was troubling: He had made calls for help when in crisis in 2010 and 2012, after which he was hospitalized. At one point, he said he wanted a SWAT team to come to kill him, in part to make him famous. Reports suggest he was chronically suicidal, suffered from depression, had obsessive-compulsive disorder, and heavily abused alcohol (Bamforth, 2014).

Life Challenges: Academic, Financial, and Familial Matters

If one must deal with mental health deficits, but has access to academic, financial, and familial supports—and if one is willing to tap into those assets—then a balance in favor of life (in terms of suicide and homicide) may be found. However, for many of the 14 figures discussed, there were also deficits of an academic, financial, and familial nature. Let us once more chronicle what is known:

1. *Jason Hamilton*: Hamilton had academic difficulty—specifically, problems with mathematics. We do not know if there were financial or family issues (Barakat, 2011).

2. *Amy Bishop*: Bishop had an intact nuclear family of a husband and two children (one of whom was actually a continuing student at the University of Alabama in Huntsville). She also had parents who were devoted to her. However, she was the primary breadwinner for her own family; her husband's earnings were helpful, but distinctly secondary in the family budget. Moreover, the loss of tenure had an academic as well as financial side: For the daughter of a college professor, and for one who had earned a PhD at Harvard, the loss of tenure could be read as academic failure (Keefe, 2013).

3. *Colton Tooley*: Tooley appears to have had no academic, financial, or family problems, but we also know very little about him. His Facebook account revealed almost nothing, and because he committed suicide there will not be court proceedings to shed much light on these three factors (CNN Wire Staff, 2010).

4. *Jared Loughner*: He had many life challenges. Published material suggests he had not done well in his classes, he had clashed with instructors, and he had been suspended (Billeaud & Tang, 2011). He dropped out of high school, had been turned down for military service, and had difficulty holding even entry-level, part-time jobs, meaning that his financial prospects were extremely limited. In fact, he survived largely by living in his parents' house and relying on them for spending money. His parents tried to help, in their fashion, such as by taking away a gun and disabling his car in the evenings so he would be less likely to get into trouble (Martinez & Carter, 2013). However, they did not help him to obtain mental health care—which officials at Pima Community

College had recommended—in part because they did not understand what was involved or how to go about it.

5. *Ross Ashley*: Comments from friends suggest that Ashley had experienced some family conflicts, but the family has been silent and the suicide essentially closed the case, so we do not know much about familial matters or about academic or financial challenges (Guarino, 2011).

6. *One L. Goh*: Goh was divorced; had lost touch with his daughter, who lived on the East Coast; and had watched his small construction company fold (Gafni, Peele, Melvin, & Krupnick, 2012). He moved from Virginia to California to get a new start, but he had heavy personal and student-related debt and few associates. His older brother and mother had recently died. Further, he was not doing well in school (Collins, 2012).

7. *James Holmes*: Holmes had a good, stable family system; he came from a family that was relatively well off, with a father who was a software engineer and a mother who was a nurse. Both parents and his sister stood by him even after the massacre. It was reported that Holmes was adopted, but it is not clear if that is accurate (Ferner, 2013). Holmes, a church-going young man who had worked as a camp counselor in summers, but who later identified as agnostic, also seemed to show promise; he had graduated from the University of California, Riverside, in 2010 with a very strong GPA, and he was a member of the Golden Key International Honour Society and the Phi Beta Kappa Society. In 2011, he gained admittance to two PhD programs. However, there were signs of difficulty. He won a prestigious internship with the Salk Institute in 2006, but his supervisor was highly critical of his performance; when he graduated from university he had trouble finding a job and apparently worked part-time at McDonald's (Delaney, 2012). Then, in 2012, his academic performance sharply deteriorated and he failed an important oral exam. Although he was not technically dismissed from the program, his lack of progress would at least have placed him on probation, and his professors encouraged him to look at other fields, which led to his resignation (Sussman, 2012). This may have been especially difficult because Holmes's father had succeeded at three prestigious schools: UCLA, UC Berkeley, and Stanford. In terms

of financial prospects, the academic outcome represented a kind of firing; Holmes naturally would not continue to receive a scholarship and stipend. His financial situation was exacerbated by the significant amounts of money he spent on guns and chemicals to make weapons ($15,000) and on prostitutes (Sussman, 2012). Finally, a number of students did reach out to him, but he was very reticent and incapable of making a connection with them. They viewed him as shy, awkward, and a loner, but they tried to help.

8. *Adam Lanza*: Lanza drove away his father and his brother repeatedly. His mother heroically tried to assist him and, in the end, sacrificed her own life to no good end. Some of the things that she tried—like sharing an interest in guns and possibly in limiting medical interventions—backfired. Lanza had no financial prospects; he was not able even to contribute to his own financial upkeep. His dream career—being a Marine—was impossible because he could not bear to be touched. Finally, he was an average but not strong student; he found introductory classes at Western Connecticut State somewhat challenging (Goldstein, 2013).

9. *James Seevakumaran*: Seevakumaran had conflicted feelings about his family. He corresponded with a prison inmate in Texas who had slain his own mother and father. After Seevakumaran passed away, his parents issued a terse statement, calling him a loner. Financially, Seevakumaran had grandiose expectations: He had had a personal goal of being a millionaire by 30; but as he entered his third decade he had significant personal and student loan debt. Further, he was about to be expelled from housing for nonpayment of rent. Academically, he had done poorly; he was not close to graduation (Davis, 2013).

10. *Dylan Quick*: We do not know of any academic, financial, or family issues that may have affected him.[15]

11. *Neil MacInnis*: His family was supportive, but we do not know of academic or economic stressors (Stevenson, n.d.).

12. *John Zawahri*: Family dynamics in Zawahri's house were complicated and conflicted. His father battered his mother, and Zawahri was upset by their divorce. Further, his father had threatened to kill his mother and the children on different occasions. Zawahri was killed by police as part of the firefight he initiated, so new

information will not emerge from court proceedings (Brown, 2013).

13. *Elliot Rodger*: Rodger attended three community colleges, but made little progress as he repeatedly dropped courses (typically because he could not abide the sight of happy romantic couples in class). He was not able or inclined to work. His plan for economic independence involved buying a sufficient number of tickets to win a Powerball lottery. His parents, stepparents, counselors, and life coaches tried to assist, but he was impervious to help (Launer, 2014).

14. *Aaron Ybarra*: Ybarra was raised in a household that seemed disordered and in which there may have been substance abuse. He was not a good student, and he was not able to support himself (Baker, 2014).

Overall View of the 14

The overall picture that emerges is of 14 individuals in truly enormous need in a number of dimensions.

First, and from a moral point of view, we are not talking about moral relativists, moral absolutists, or moral realists. We are talking about people, for the most part, who think and act in a way that is immoral or, more likely, morally vacant. The cases put one face-to-face with organic nihilism, which rejects moral and ethical principles and takes the position that life is meaningless. Or to put it another way, life can be seen as just a cosmic video game, and all its citizens potential casualties. The absence of feeling for the sanctity of life, the fascination with truly perverse things, the utter lack of pity, and a range of emotions that runs from rage to indifference but never to love—it is rather breathtaking.

Second, from a psychological point of view, we are dealing with very serious mental health conditions. Paranoid schizophrenia and mania that leads to psychosis, for example, constitute two very large challenges. Even our best pharmacological aids have value only if those needing to take them are willing to do so. Unfortunately, as we have seen in cases ranging from Cho to Ybarra, this is frequently not the case. To be sure, we are not dealing with relatively easy-to-assist students—such as those contending with test anxiety or a first romantic breakup—who will find short-term counseling of great assistance. We are dealing with people who need close social supervision, if not hospitalization.

Third, many of these individuals have serious deficits of an academic, familial, or financial nature, and significant life pressures tend to reinforce moral and psychological challenges. And it can be difficult to remedy these individual deficits for larger reasons. To that point, concerns about limited financial aid and accumulating student loan debt pertain to not only Goh or Loughner but also millions of students. In addition, families cannot always provide the breadth and depth of support that a very troubled young adult may need, even when they try hard, as was the tragic case with Nancy Lanza, Adam Lanza's mother. And to maintain academic integrity, grades and degrees cannot be provided to mollify, appease, or encourage a troubled person like Holmes. Although a measure of leniency and an occasional academic break can be helpful and beneficial, degrees need to be awarded for quality intellectual work (earned through coursework) or for extraordinary societal accomplishment (the honorary degree), not to provide a placebo effect.

Fourth, by and large, these are not people who had been misused or bullied by their communities. More often than not, these are people who had misused or bullied their own communities. So if there is a moral duty to help, there is an even greater moral duty to help them to help themselves. Otherwise, we find ourselves supporting the meanest and most exploitative form of entitlement.

A Final Observation on Rampage Shootings — Permeability

The subject of this first section has been rampage shooters and shootings that have significant ties with academe. However, we should remember that such events are not restricted to institutions of higher education. One can easily document rampage shootings that have taken place over the last 30 years in high schools, middle schools, elementary schools, and religious schools. And off-campus rampage shootings in the same period have occurred at least once in each of the following venues: brokerage houses, city halls, churches, commercial cafeterias, county offices, fast-food restaurants, immigration centers, Italian restaurants, Jewish centers, law offices, lottery offices, manufacturing plants, military bases, motels/hotels, museums, nursing homes, pancake houses, post offices, shopping malls, Sikh temples, supermarkets, and so on. And some rampage-shooting cases that combined gun and car over roadways have made the phenomenon quite mobile.[16]

Increasingly, matters are permeable. Violence can travel back and forth between on campus and off campus with some regularity. Thus, although reform-minded people must focus on violence on campus, they also ought to keep a close eye on what is happening in society as a whole.

More Conventional Homicide and Higher Education

In the Talmud, there is a saying that can be rendered, "The taking of a single life is like destroying the entire world; and the saving of a single life is like saving the entire world" (Bart, 2014). It can remind us—regardless of our highly variable religious and secular backgrounds—of the importance of dealing with not only dramatic rampage events, which can take many lives at once, but also lesser homicide incidents, which typically involve one or two victims. This is particularly important in higher education, where sexual assault, domestic violence, hazing, brawling, and drug and alcohol abuse can lead to the tragic loss of life in the full flower of youth—even if on a singular or dual rather than a mass basis. Therefore, we now turn our attention to conventional homicide.

Looking at the Clery Data

To obtain a baseline estimate of the number of faculty, students, and staff affected by homicide in academe, we turn to the Jeanne Clery Disclosure of Campus Security Policy and Campus Crime Statistics Act, 1992 (hereafter referred to as the Clery Act).[17] Clery reports, which are required by the act, track specific criminal violations, including homicide. They focus on murders that have taken place at institutions of higher education, or in their immediate environs—that is, on campus, in collegiate residence halls, in noncampus buildings of the institution, and on adjacent public property.

Data for 2013 and 2014 are not yet available. However, pertinent information is extant for 2005 and 2006 (just before our period of concern), for 2007 and 2008 (when seminal events at VT and NIU took place), and for 2009 through 2012 (in the period that is the focus of this chapter). Table 1.1 summarizes the results.[18]

For 2005 and 2006, the number of reported homicides stands in the mid- to higher 20s, or roughly 20-something too high. Pragmatically, however, these two numbers—28 and 25—are not surprising, given the millions of students enrolled at U.S. universities and colleges in the 50 states and associated territories and given the violent tenor of much of American life.

More alarming was the dramatic upturn in 2007. Sixty-six incidents represents an enormous increase, whether one looks back or ahead. However, if one deducts 33 (the loss of life experienced at VT on April 16), the resultant figure is not so very wide off the expected mark. Moreover, this anomaly does illustrate vividly the potential impact a malevolent and tactically astute rampage shooter can make: In one day and to one school such a person brought the amount of carnage that it would take thousands of universities and colleges an entire year to produce.

The result for 2008, 55, is large and puzzling. Even if one subtracts the five murdered people at NIU, the remainder of 50 still represents a significant increase. Perhaps events of 2007 and early 2008 gave some people of ill will a kind of unstated permission to act out cruelly. It is not unreasonable to assume that two highly dramatic

Table 1.1   Homicides According to Aggregated Clery Reports, 2005–2012

Year	Number of victims of homicide
2005	28
2006	25
2007	66
2008	55
2009	32
2010	33
2011	33
2012	31

Table 1.2   Number of Deaths in On-Campus Residence Halls

Year	Number of deaths
2012	5
2011	2
2010	2
2009	4

acts of violence could have produced a disinhibiting effect in some individuals.

Then matters appear to calm down as we enter a kind of plateau for 4 years. For 2009–2012 the average is 32.25, with a very narrow range of 31 to 33.

The overarching Clery data underscore the work to be done: It would be very good to lower the death rate progressively from the 30s to the 20s to the teens, and so forth. However, it does *not* appear that matters are growing worse, if Clery-reported homicides are the principal indicator.

Recent Clery reports demonstrate that university residence halls tend to be quite safe. The national death rate for students in on-campus housing accommodations was 3.25 per annum for 2009 to 2012, with a range of 2 to 5 (Table 1.2). Properly locked doors, well-trained resident assistants, a good community ethos (rooted in principles of bystander intervention), and partnerships with campus police can create safe living patterns.

These data have important implications for university administrators, taxpayers, and donors. They suggest that investment in campus housing can help create and maintain safer academic communities. Well-designed living–learning centers can not only facilitate intellectual and professional growth but also create a more peaceful and nonviolent environment, especially if such housing is provided for not only first-year students but also interested sophomores, juniors, seniors, and graduate students.

200 University Murder or Attempted Murder Cases[19]

I collected the 200 stories of university murder or attempted murder cases (mostly focused on students) from Internet searches for the period from January 2009 through June 2014, or 5.5 years. I excluded cases that involved manslaughter or gross negligence (i.e., death due to DUI, alcohol poisoning/aspiration, drug overdose, or complications with late-term abortions or self-delivered infants).

I concede that even very assiduous Internet searches cannot provide a completely random sample. It is likely that events that took place in larger markets and that featured more salacious details would be more prominently and repetitively told.

On the other hand, it is also the case that murder is an item of interest in a market of almost any size; if the story is told in only one or two outlets, that serves as well as if it were publicized in 100 features, as long as it is seen. In addition, the Internet is a place where the content of even very modest news organizations is consistently featured. And given the recent time period (no case older than 5.5 years), loss of stories (due to superannuation) would seem quite unlikely, especially as murder cases are subject to frequent updates in the early years. Therefore, I expected, and found, that the Internet accounts formed a robust resource on which to rely.

Tables 1.3 and 1.4 report the number of people involved in murder-related incidents. The results reiterate that the vast majority of murder cases do not resemble the broadest rampage incidents, which receive lots of coverage. Most homicides, in fact, involve a single victim.

Table 1.3   Murder of University People: January 2009 Through June 2014

Number of murdered	Number of incidents	Percentage of incidents
Zero (all recovered from attempted murder)	13	6.5
One	172	86.0
Two	10	5.0
Three	4	2.0
Four, five, or six	0	0.0
Seven	1	0.5
More than seven	0	0.0
Total	200	100.0

Table 1.4   Number of Casualties in 200 Incidents From January
2009 Through June 2014 (deaths and injuries)

Number of people	Number of incidents	Percentage of incidents
One	154	77.0
Two	29	14.5
Three	10	5.0
Four	3	1.5
Five	0	0.0
Six	2	1.0
Seven	0	0.0
More than seven	2	1.0
Total	200	100.0

Regarding casualties (both killings and injuries), the vast majority
of cases (91.5%) fall within the framework of one or two harmed.
And if one adds three casualties, the total rises to 96.5%.

Thus, on the basis of both fatalities and casualties, conventional
crime is the much more ominous threat. The larger rampage killing
cases are frightening and serious—especially if they increase—but
the frequency should still not be exaggerated.

Causation and Type

The most often seen type of crime (46.5%) involved common or street
crime: theft; mugging; fights; gang-related activity; and escalating
conflict among strangers, acquaintances, and friends (Table 1.5).

For example, in April 2010, Vincent Binder, a graduate student
at Florida State University, was stabbed and robbed off campus by
Quenton Truehill, an escaped convict (Korfage, 2014). Substance-
related crimes were also not infrequent. As a case in point, Max
Moreno, a student at Pace University, was killed by Raymond Rizzo
and an associate in a search for drugs in September 2010 (Baker,
2010). Stephen Johnson, of Temple University, died in January, 2013
in the aftermath of a fight that began at a party ("Arrest Made,"
2013).

Table 1.5   Types of Crimes Associated With Homicide

Type	Number	Percentage
Common/street crime	93	46.5
Domestic conflicts	37	18.5
Predatory sexual crime	16	8.0
Impulsive killing	9	4.5
Suicidal linked	7	3.5
Workplace conflict	7	3.5
Familial killings	5	2.5
Drug psychosis	3	1.5
Extreme gun negligence, but no intent to harm	3	1.5
Political, helping bystanders, financial, hazing	8 (2 each)	4.0
Unknown	12	6.0
Total	200	100.0

Domestic conflicts were also relatively common, seen in 18.5% of cases. One might mention the particularly sad case of a young female student, Emily Silverstein, of Gettysburg College, who was killed by her ex-boyfriend, Kevin Schaeffer (also a student at Gettysburg College), who was said to have self-medicated with marijuana and alcohol rather than with antidepressants (Herman, 2010).

Predatory sexual conduct (8%) involved very dark cases where aggravated assault and perverse exploitation were found. The targeted included both straight and gay, female and male, and Craigslist misuse was mentioned twice. The interaction frequently occurred among strangers or virtual strangers. A particularly stark case involved Seth Mazzaglia and Kathryn McDonough, who, in late June 2014, were sentenced to life and 15 years in prison, respectively, for having kidnapped, enslaved, repeatedly violated, and killed a 19-year-old University of New Hampshire female student (Tuohy, 2014).

I had not expected an impulsive urge to kill to be a factor, but it was a significant contributing factor in many instances. For example,

John Shaffer, a 20-year-old student at the University of Texas at Dallas, cut the throat of his female teaching assistant—whom he hardly knew—because he felt an overwhelming, inexplicable impulse to harm (Jennings, 2010). Similarly, Jerrod Murray, of East Central University in Oklahoma, murdered Gennaro Sanchez off campus because he wanted to know what it felt like to kill a human being. Murray reassured authorities afterward that he had nothing personal against Sanchez (Morava, 2013).

At 3.5% were people who placed themselves in situations that involved murder or attempted murder in large part to bring about suicide. Consider, for example, the case of Odane Greg Maye, a student who had not been academically successful at Hampton University, and who had departed. Returning to his on-campus residence hall in April 2009 while carrying three guns, he wounded a building monitor and a pizza deliveryman. Newspaper accounts shared that Maye suffered from depression, bipolar disorder, and schizophrenia, and in his writings he expressed a desire to end it all. Maye was wounded and survived; he was sentenced to 14 years in prison (Dujardin, 2009).

Workplace conflict occurred at different levels. Previously, I discussed Amy Bishop, who shot faculty colleagues. In March 2010, in a more narrowly targeted event, Nathaniel Brown, a custodian at Ohio State, shot two other staff members, including his supervisor, due to dissatisfaction with work-performance ratings ("Suspect Kills," 2010). And at SUNY–Binghampton, Abdulsalam al-Zahrani, a graduate student, fatally stabbed his adviser, in part because he felt that the professor was plotting against him (this also might be seen as an example of a politically motivated killing) ("Abdulsalam al-Zahrani," 2011).

Location

Table 1.6, covering 2009 to 2014, confirms what we had suggested when reviewing this same matter several years ago (Ferraro & McHugh, 2010): Campus living tends to be much safer than off-campus alternatives (these data suggest an approximate increased safety ratio of 3.5 to 1), even when on- and off-campus living share the same city, town, or neighborhood.

Table 1.6   Locations of University-Related Murders or Attempted
Murders From 2009 to 2014

Location of pertinent incidents	Number	Percentage
On campus (residence halls, academic buildings, university parking lots, etc.)	42	21.0
Off campus (off-campus residences, houses, restaurants, stores, bars, etc.)	145	72.5
Remote locations (internships, vacations, breaks, visiting friends out of town, study abroad, etc.)	13	6.5
Total	200	100.0

I included the remote living category to indicate that students, leading complicated lives, sometimes fall prey to death or injury while they are studying abroad, on internships, on vacation, at home, and so on. Although it is hard to make a meaningful risk comparison between on-campus living and remote living (in part because the latter constitutes only a relatively small portion of a student's collegiate career and is so varied), the point can be extracted that even going home on vacation is no guarantee of safety.

On-campus living tends to be quite safe for several reasons, including capable housing staff and resident assistants, a sense of knowing and being known (not being anonymous), threat assessment and care teams, skilled community policing, high community standards, and proximal counseling centers.

All this notwithstanding, when there is a murder on campus, there is profound disappointment because all—parents, faculty, students, and staff—want to believe that universities can be safe havens, sanctuaries in a violent society.

Victims and Gender

Table 1.7 shows the breakdown of murder victims by biological sex.

On first glance, it is not surprising that a greater number of males run the risk of murder in comparison with females, especially given

Table 1.7   Sex of Murdered People (200 Cases and 250 People)

Sex	Number killed or injured	Percentage
Female	90	36.0
Male	160	64.0
Total	250	100.0

the impact of common or street crime, which is well represented in the data and which can affect men disproportionately. However, the degree of difference is still surprising, especially when male university enrollment nationally is closer to 40% than 50%.

As might be assumed, the data show that women are most often victimized with respect to domestic violence. In only 4 of 37 cases was the female the murderer. Of those cases, three victims were male and one was female.

Perpetrators of Murder and Gender

As might be expected—and likely for both biological and sociological reasons—women appear much less likely than men to commit or to contribute to murder. In fact, on the basis of our collected data, females make up slightly more than 10% of the known and responsible population (Table 1.8).

Turning from quantitative to qualitative aspects, I had expected the women in our data list to play a not insignificant but largely indirect role. For example, in May 2009, Brittany Smith, a Harvard University student, helped her boyfriend commit a robbery in a university residence hall that led to the killing of a drug dealer. It was she who provided ID entry, who helped lure the victim, and who tried to hide the weapon after the fact; so she bore important responsibility. However, she did not pull the trigger (Yu, 2011). Nonetheless, in the collected data, on at least some occasions, women played a direct role.

For example, in October 2013, Sparkles Lashayla Lindsey became involved in an incident of road rage with Kimberly Faith Kilgore, a student at Kennesaw State University. Lindsey followed Kilgore into her off-campus, gated community, pulled out a gun, and shot the 21-year-old student to death (Gorman, 2014).

Table 1.8   Sex of People Who Murdered or Attempted to Murder (200 Cases and 269 People)

Sex	Number who killed or seriously injured	Percentage
Female	27	10.04
Male	222	82.53
Unknown	20	7.43
Total	269	100.0

Shayna Hubers, a student in a master's program in counseling at Eastern Kentucky University, exhibited an ice-cold indifference more befitting a male figure in an Elmore Leonard novel than the cultural expectations Americans generally hold for women. Using one of three guns the couple kept in the apartment for protection, after she and her significant other had had a purely verbal altercation at the kitchen table, Hubers shot her lawyer boyfriend twice in the face—later sardonically saying that she finally gave him the nose job that he always wanted. She then shot him four more times because she found the twitching of his body disquieting (Farberov & Golgowski, 2012).

Andrea Nicole Alvira did not even need a weapon. This 19-year-old escort had verbally contracted with and provided a sexual service for Brandon Day, a 22-year-old student at Palm Beach State University. When Day refused to pay, and so committed a kind of theft of service, she tackled him and then suffocated him to death by pressing her knee on his neck ("Female Escort," 2014).

Do these cases suggest that violence among women is likely to sharply increase in the future? I do not believe so. The cases are limited and fragmented, but they do underscore that violence is not an exclusive province of men.

Instruments of Death

Table 1.9 gives a breakdown of instruments of death used in murders from 2009 to 2014.

In nearly 60% of these murders, guns were the key instrument of death. Of handguns used, semiautomatics were much more

Table 1.9 Weapons Used in Murders or in Attempted Murders
(January 2009–June 2014)

Type of weapon	Number	Percentage
Gun	123	59.13
Stabbing (principally by knife)	36	15.87
Strangulation or suffocation	22	10.58
Blunt force trauma	18	8.65
Car (used as a weapon)	4	1.92
Unknown (reason unclear or information not released)	5	2.40
Total	208*	100.0

*Note. More than one type of weapon may have been used in an incident or with different persons.

common; revolvers have become rather antiquated. We also frequently saw extended clips. There were also some assault and conventional rifles and shotguns. There were no automatic weapons, such as light machine guns, in the data.

Stabbing was the next most common means of killing, with knives being the principal instrument employed. We did, however, also note grave wounds inflicted by scissors and a hatchet. Three people carried, but likely did not fatally employ, a sword and two machetes. Knives were also not infrequently found as auxiliary weapons, to be carried along with a rifle or handgun.

Strangulation was the third most common means of killing, found frequently in domestic conflicts and predatory sexual assault cases. It included suffocation caused by rope, hands, or forced drowning.

Blunt force trauma caused 18 deaths. Pertinent objects included fists, a baseball bat, a metal pipe, a hammer, and a dumbbell. Being stomped to death and being repeatedly tackled (during hazing) also played a role. And one student was permanently felled by the "punch-out game," a hopefully outdated fad in which a tough would knock out a passing pedestrian with a sucker punch, usually to win a bet. In this particular case a wager cost one young man his academic career and the other 10 years in prison. Blunt force trauma tended to be associated with street and bar fights and impulsive clashes.

We mentioned earlier that DUI deaths were not incorporated into this study, but cars were involved in several fatalities when used purposefully to strike people or when people were thrown into the automobile's path.

Individuals who oppose gun regulation frequently say that if there were no guns or even just fewer guns, people would still kill each other with knives, baseball bats, chains, or crowbars. While there is some truth in this, a gun-free or gun-restricted environment would certainly reduce the speed, ease, and lethality of murder. In addition, it likely would convert more murders into attempted murders, as injured people would have a greater chance of recovering in the hospital.

Blunt force trauma and strangulation are not suited for rampage killing. They just do not kill sufficiently quickly or efficiently to serve. And we also should remember that many of the rampage killers were not imposing physical figures: Cho had a scrawny physique, and Lanza stood 6 feet tall, but weighed 112 pounds. A would-be killer might be successfully thwarted if he or she relied on Stone Age weapons.

Knives can be quite lethal. In the nineteenth century, the bowie knife was banned or restricted in many jurisdictions because of its potential as a deadly man-killer. And there are a few collegiate cases in which knives exacted a heavy toll. We mentioned previously the example from Lone Star Community College in April 2013, during which a student injured 14 peers—but killed none—with a scalpel and an X-Acto knife. Then, in May 2014, Elliot Rodger, a student at Santa Barbara City College, killed three roommates (students at UC–Santa Barbara) with a hammer and knives. The most lethal knife attack in a college setting occurred recently just outside of the geographical scope of this study (in Canada); however, I mention it here to illustrate what might be viewed as the end of the lethal range.

Early one morning in April 2014, Matthew de Grood, a student at the University of Calgary and an invited guest to a house party of some 30 University of Calgary students, killed five schoolmates (four men and one woman) with two knives (one he brought and one he stole from the house). Three students expired quickly due to critically placed wounds, and two others died at the hospital the next day. Not all details have been released, but it appears that de Grood was successful because he managed to isolate the five people, one at time, in separate rooms in their common house. Alcohol may have limited alertness and delayed defensive reactions (Canadian Press, 2014).

All in all, a knife is a serious weapon, but it does not seem well placed to create a heavy death toll in most circumstances. For this reason, semiautomatic guns are the weapons of choice.

Murder, Race, and Ethnicity

Finally, as I was collecting data on murders, I recorded information that was easy to find on race and ethnicity with the intent of learning more about possible hate crimes, especially those that might result in fatalities.

Whether racism directly caused murders remained unclear. I did not find cases that pointed to overt racism as the progenitor of actual murder. Instead, I confirmed that murderous incidents, especially if perpetrator and victim were of different races, tended to bring out the worst in human thought and expression.

The brutal Channon Christian and Christopher Newsom rape-murders of 2007, for example, continued to generate an abundance of racial animus on one side and a seeming lack of sympathy for the victims of a truly terrible crime on the other (Jones, 2012).

There was one finding that was interesting and had to do with the racial disproportion seen in victims of murder—even in the context of presumably more privileged college students (Table 1.10).

The number of slain Caucasians is the highest of any group, with 95 entries. However, Caucasians also represent the largest group in

Table 1.10 Murder Victims' Race and Ethnicity

Ethnicity	Number	Percentage
African or African American	85	34.0
Asian (East, Central, and Near Eastern)	28	11.2
Hispanic	11	4.4
Native American	1	0.4
White	95	38.0
Unknown	30	12.0
Total	250	100.0

society. The number of Native Americans is low (only one death), but that is not surprising because the number of indigenous people on campuses across the country is equally low.

For African Americans, the number is disproportionately high. The data collected show 85 entries, or 34% of the total, and the situation is even more skewed for African American males (76 deaths).

This is one small datum in a relatively small data set, and I do not want to exaggerate the finding. However, if diversity is to be taken seriously, it surely means that African American men on campus should find not only an invigorating intellectual environment but also a secure physical home. And if we are serious about promoting a new generation of male leaders, security has to be a *sine qua non* condition.

The Picture at Community Colleges

Few community colleges offer on-campus student housing, so the aspect of the Clery Act that relates to homicides in college-owned dormitories or residence halls is largely irrelevant. However, other categories found in Clery (the campus, affiliated buildings off campus, and adjacent public space) are pertinent. By patching together separate reports extracted from Clery, we can offer the overview in Table 1.11 on frequency of homicides specific to public community colleges from 2009–2012.

All in all, 16% to 21% of homicide cases that took place in these 4 years involved public community colleges. Most of these were related activity on adjacent public space.

Table 1.11   **Number of Homicides at Public Community Colleges**

Year	Number of homicides at public community colleges	Percentage of homicides occurring at all postsecondary institutions
2009	6	18.75
2010	7	21.21
2011	6	18.18
2012	5	16.13
2009–2012	24	18.60

The careful reader may note that I did not include tallies of private community colleges or junior colleges in Table 1.11. The reason for that exclusion is purely technical. The pertinent group was too small to allow extraction from Clery on a state-by-state basis and obtain a comparable subtotal.

50 Community College Murder or Attempted Murder Cases

We saw that universities and community colleges were fairly equally touched by the threat of rampage shooters. By and large, a common pattern is seen when we turn to conventional murder demonstrated by the 50 community college cases that we reviewed (extracted from Internet sources).

Lethality of Incidents

Beginning with the lethality of incidents, in these 50 events of murder or attempted murder at community colleges in the period under review (2009–2014), one- and two-person murders were most common. More specifically, 7 events involved no deaths (people recovered from attempted murder), 33 cases involved a single death, 5 cases involved 2 deaths, and 2 cases involved 2 deaths. However, in two events, losses were quite large: 5 and 6 dead.

If we turn to casualties (death and injuries), 72% of cases involved harm to two or fewer people; in nine cases (18%), three people were killed or wounded. In two cases, four and six people counted as casualties. Finally, there were three events that qualified as very high-casualty: 10, 14, and 20.

Types of Homicide Cases

The breakdown by type of homicide for community college students once more is led by common or street crime (23 cases), including robbery, gang violence, drug-related deals, and drive-by shootings.

Domestic conflict is also commonly seen (nine cases), mostly focused on the unwillingness of involved males to accept the decision of a female partner to end a relationship. Such was the case involving John Darrel Theusen, of Blinn College, in March 2009 ("Conviction," 2014); Robert J. Vaughan, of Broward College, in May 2009 (Santana & Nolin, 2009); and Jonathan Pena Castillo, of Bronx Community College, in January 2013 (Kemp, Hutchinson, & Cunningham, 2013). The case of Daniel Wilyam, of the Art Institute of Dallas, was a variation of the theme: He killed a female student in September 2009 for indirect reasons, or because he saw her as a potential rival for the affections of a young man (Goldstein, 2011). Tiaunna Hall stabbed her live-in boyfriend, Anthony Martemus, of Cuyahoga Community College, in the heart (Shaffer, 2014).

Predatory sexual crime included five cases. In one case the rage was rooted in a domestic breakup, which led to the brutal rape and murder of Rita Morelli, an international student at Manhattan Community College, by Bakary Camara, another international student at the same school, in November 2011 (Parascandola & Kemp, 2011). Still the most difficult case to read was one involving the rape/strangulation of a girl who had barely passed her 10th birthday, committed by Austin Sigg, an 18-year-old student at Arapahoe Community College, with strong interests in pornography and mortuary science (Steffen, 2013).

We also saw five instances of familicide, the most noteworthy of which concerned Professor James Krumm, of Casper Community College. This dedicated teacher was slain by his son, Christopher Krumm, who shot him with a bow and arrow. Krumm also killed his father's common-law wife and himself with a knife (Gruver, 2012).

Suicidal desire expressed itself in three events, and three cases might fairly reflect a strong desire to kill.

In four cases, we suggest the cause might be academic frustration, being in the wrong place at the wrong time (a fallen bystander), financial distress, and unknown.

Finally, a very interesting case of drug psychosis might be mentioned. Joshua Davis, aged 32, was smoking marijuana with three younger friends who attended Polk State College in Florida. After a short while he began to get a "dark feeling" (Little, 2012), and then he experienced an overwhelming but totally misplaced fear that the three students were plotting to kill his baby daughter. Arming himself with a gun, he executed two of them while wounding the third, committing this mayhem in front of his small child (Little, 2012).

Location and Relative Safety

With community college students, as with university students, danger is much more likely to happen off campus than on campus. Murders or attempted murders occurred on campus or its environs 22% of the time, whereas off campus the percentage rose to 70%. In our sample of 50 incidents, students died in remote locations in 4 cases (8%).

Gender of Victims

In keeping with what we found for university students, in this sample of 50 incidents and 86 identified people, collegiate males faced a disproportionate chance of being a murder victim. However, the gap between men and women was narrower (less than 13 percentage points) than with university students for reasons that are not entirely clear.

In the data there was one transgender victim noted (a 19-year-old student of Spartanburg Community College), who was stabbed 22 times and shot twice in the head by Sama Chaka Quinland. Quinland claimed that he acted out of uncontrolled rage when he discovered that the student "was a man rather than a woman" as they engaged each other sexually. The court assigned a sentence of 30 years in prison, in part because of the great brutality of the murder, but also because Quinland had committed theft, tried to elude police, and had at least one prior arrest (Kimzey, 2013).

Gender of Murderers

Of identifiable people, the percentage of females was 9.26% (similar to that found for university students, at 10.4%). As for males, once more based on identified perpetrators, the percentage was 90.74%. In six cases it was not possible to identify the sex of the offending individual.

Weaponry Used (50 Incidents Using 61 Items)

Once more, guns were the favored instruments for murder (used in 38 cases, or 62.29%). Most guns were handguns, but a few shotguns and rifles were employed. In keeping with what was seen with university students, among community college students, stabbing was the next most common means of murder (12, or 19.67%). Again, knives were the most common instrument for stabbing. In four cases each, strangulation or suffocation was used (6.56% each). And these killing methods were used one time each: bow and arrow, striking with an automobile, and throwing a person under a train.

This brief review of community college cases confirms that when it comes to issues of safety and security—especially at the level of homicide—they are not very different from issues at universities.

Reforms to Make for a Better and Safer Future

Rampage shootings are not common at U.S. colleges and universities, and they do not affect a large percentage of students, faculty, and staff, even indirectly. However, when they occur, they have the capacity to create appalling damage in human and institutional terms, which can not only unsettle a university and its environs but also ripple through a state and even demoralize a nation. Further, it seems clear that these rampage events are occurring more frequently than in the past, which is a source of deep concern. Qualitatively, the rampage incidents discussed in this chapter range from terrible to truly horrific.

Further, we also must not lose sight of "conventional" homicide, which may be less widely publicized, but which can have a profound impact on individuals, families, friends, the school, and the wider community. Qualitatively, what unfolds in some fatal domestic conflicts and with predatory sexual behavior can rival rampage events in terms of ferocity and baseness.

People can become passive in the face of killing crimes because they cynically chalk it up to living in a violent society. Moreover, violence, especially gun violence, is part of the fabric of American life. A 2013 study by Dr. Sripal Bangalore, of NYU Langone Medical Center, and Dr. Franz Messerli, of St. Luke's Medical Center, noted that the United States ranked first in guns and gun deaths among 27 developed countries (with 88 guns per 100 people and 10.2 gun deaths per 100,000 people). In contrast, the figures for Canada were 30.8 guns per 100 people and 2.44 gun deaths per 100,000 people (Leahy, 2013).

The fact that gun violence is prevalent, however, should not be a reason for passivity; it should be a call to action. Even if we cannot totally eliminate gun violence, there is much room for improvement.

Sensible Gun Policies and Practices

A logical place to start reducing violence is with gun policies and practices. I drew up a policy statement on guns on campus for the Enough Is Enough campaign, which was later largely adopted by NASPA–Student Affairs Administrators in Higher Education, to my deep appreciation. This civil and reasoned policy statement shows respect for the interests of hunters in the field, for those who need to defend person and property *in their own homes*, and for those moved by intellectual curiosity (e.g., the Civil War reenactor with period arms). But it takes the position that guns do not belong on campus, save in the hands of campus police or for related degree programming, such as military officer training. This stand was taken for several reasons:

> ➤ Disputes, especially on campuses of higher education, should be settled by research, writing, and debate, not by force or armed intimidation.
> ➤ The presence of guns is inconsistent with suicide prevention, and this demands attention as university and college students have a relatively high incidence of suicidal ideation.
> ➤ Guns on campus constitute an enhanced risk because university and college students tend to consume alcohol more immoderately than other age groups.
> ➤ Safe storage of guns is almost an oxymoron given the close and communal living conditions found in most residence halls.
> ➤ A no-gun policy conforms to what is done in all other types of educational institutions, including high schools.

> It is unlikely that an untrained militia (students or faculty carrying weapons by virtue of "open carry," "concealed carry," or "constitutional carry") could safely defuse rampage events. In fact, due to factors like friendly fire, panic fire, ricochet fire, inaccurate fire, misdirected fire, and frozen fire, it is likely that armed and untrained or lightly trained students or faculty would seriously inflate casualties and make rampage events even deadlier.

The aforementioned Enough Is Enough policy document provides a logical basis for gun-free campuses, and it inserts compassion and dispassion into a debate that is too often driven by passion. It reminds us that a peaceful approach has merit. It helps universities and colleges retain the ideal of a safe haven.

Given what we have seen about permeability, however, is the campus perspective enough? In incidents that took place recently in Santa Monica and Santa Barbara, we saw rampages that crossed borders between simply on and off campus. James Holmes and Jared Loughner—counseled and appropriately suspended from the university and college, respectively—directed their heated anger at a movie theater and a shopping center (where they killed or injured 90 people).

Right-Sizing Counseling Center Services

Traditionally, university counseling centers have featured short-term and limited treatment, focused on the following goals: (a) supporting the academic mission, (b) enhancing student growth and development, and (c) dealing with short-term crises. The more critical cases and those that involve heavy user services might well be referred off campus.

Today, these missions are still relevant, but others can be added: (d) managing chronic (and sometimes severe) mental health conditions, and (e) conducting threat assessment. In addition, although service today is still frequently short term, it can also involve intermediate or long-term variations. Referring very serious cases or those interested in regular and frequent sessions to off-campus resources can make sense, but it has to be balanced with the oversight needed for good threat assessment.

The traditional recommended level of staffing for psychological care at universities has been one counselor for every 1,000–1,500 students, a standard that many universities for financial reasons do not reach, even if we are talking about the upper end of the range. However, given the extraordinary needs of the students described in this chapter, one might argue that a ratio of 1:1,000 or 1:1,200 should be implemented.

Given their traditional missions, many community colleges do not have counseling centers. In some states, in fact, they are instructed not to provide mental health services. However, 7 of 14 rampage shooters were community college students, and in the data on more conventional homicides, there are certainly a number of people from 2-year schools who could have benefited from sophisticated psychological services. Therefore, it would be good if community colleges were given sufficient resources so that they could offer at least a modicum of services in this area.

In addition, given the role of psychotropic drugs, and the importance of medication management, it is important for universities and desirable for community colleges to offer psychiatric services.

The contradiction, of course, resides with funding and staffing. Most students, parents, and government officials want to have additional or new mental health services, but they are all concerned about keeping the cost of attendance low. However, if the human costs associated with rampage violence and with conventional violence are weighed, investment in mental health services justifies itself.

Therefore, if universities can right-size their counseling staffs—that is, take into account what is needed for the breadth and depth of service—and if community colleges can acquire a modicum of pertinent offerings, that would increase safety and make for healthier minds. Even incremental improvement has value.

Suicide, Homicide, Title II, and Involuntary Leave

Most students who experience passing suicidal thoughts can be well cared for on campus. Many students who have a growing preoccupation with suicide, have seriously thought about how they might end their lives, or have made a legitimate attempt to commit suicide might also successfully cope—with help and support—and successfully remain on campus. Yet, there are some students who are strongly suicidal and for whom suicidality occurs with homicidality. These people have to be looked at more closely on a case-by-case basis. The Americans with Disabilities Act is not an excuse for a lack of critical thinking about risk in this area, especially when suicide, although correlated with depression, is not in itself a mental health condition.

It is true that most people who are suicidal are not homicidal. However, if one reviews the 14 rampage killers listed in this study, at least 10 thought about, attempted, or completed suicide before, during, or after the incident. It is not illogical to assume that a person who is willing to take his or her own life might not have strong reverence for the lives of others.

For many years both universities and the federal government agreed that people who represented direct threats to themselves (suicide) or others (homicide) could be required to interrupt their education without violating federal antidiscrimination law. Involuntary withdrawal from school was intended to give the person in crisis time, space, and incentive for recovery, and it generally foresaw a return to studies. However, in 2011, a reinterpretation of Title II preserved the right of the university to take action if there were direct threats to others, but it omitted reference to direct threats to self, raising many questions and presenting many contradictions (Grasgreen, 2014).[20]

The 2011 reinterpretation, however, did not require the suicidal individual to cooperate in the least with people in authority who are trying to offer help. This lack of personal self-help inevitably shifts responsibility without authority to the school and its help-givers—almost a perfect definition of *burdensomeness*.

In addition, the distinction between harm to self and harm to others breaks down when one thinks of people like the killers at Columbine, VT, NIU, Central Florida, Sandy Hook, Santa Barbara, and so on, who embodied both suicidal and homicidal aspects, even if the latter was fully apparent only after the fact. One might argue that too liberal concessions made to suicide elevate the danger of homicide.

There would be many humanitarian and material advantages if the federal government returned to the pre-2011 standard, where due weight was given to both direct threat to self and direct threat to others. One could provide protection for students who may be contemplating suicide but who do not pose a strong direct threat to themselves by including a number of salient protections:

> ➢ Require that all people who are reviewed for involuntary leave receive individualized consideration and qualified assessment. Involuntary leave should be part of an individualized therapeutic package for students who register severe concerns. It should not be a means to summarily remove students with complicated lives.
> ➢ Require that all involuntary leaves be temporary (i.e., last no more than a semester or year). Involuntary leave should be the pause that allows the person in crisis to return to studies with a renewed chance for personal and academic success.
> ➢ Require a treatment plan at departure that sketches out fully what the student reasonably has to do to return, so that the time away can and will be used to good effect and misunderstandings can be minimized.

All in all, involuntary medical leave is a useful tool as long as it is used with fairness and restraint. It also can be a way to reduce damage related to suicide/homicide. If the U.S. Department of Education's Office for Civil Rights could return to pre-2011 days, it would help make safer campuses.

Conclusion

We began this chapter with the man who made himself an island, Seung-Hui Cho, a man who betrayed his classmates, his parents, his school, and his new country on April 16, 2007, for no comprehensible reason; a man who surely was mad, not only because of his mental state but also because he embodied so much wrath. But the tragedy of that day had less to do with the crime of the shooter and much more to do with the loss of 32 beautiful, talented, and diverse people who were taken from families, friends, and colleagues too soon and in such a bitter way.

As we end this chapter, although acknowledging the importance of the vast amount of data shared within, we should turn for a final moment and reflect on the human element. Specifically, we turn to May 23, 2014, more than 7 years after the incident at VT, to the day on which Rodger, a version of Cho, in the unincorporated community near Santa Barbara, California, called Isla Vista, shot Bianca de Kock, a member of Tri Delta (Vega, Gard, Vojtech, Keohane, & Berardi, 2014). He fatally shot two of her sorority sisters, and then— after smiling at her—he shot her five times.

Why do we do what we do to try to stem the tide of violence? Ultimately, it is very simple. It is to try to ensure our students' safety.

Notes

1. Sometimes a "conventional crime" can produce high casualties. For example, Columbus Jones and Braylon Rogers, unhappy about being excluded from an off-campus fraternity party at Youngstown University, returned with loaded guns and killed an individual and wounded 11 others (Dick, 2011).

2. The 1966 rampage shooting by Charles Whitman at the University of Texas at Austin involved dual siting (at his home and then at the bell tower on campus); in 2007, Seung-Hui Cho killed two people in a residence hall near his own dormitory and then committed many murders in a classroom building across campus. We also note the shootings of John Zawahri and Elliot Rodger, which involved triple siting: at home, on campus, and on town streets.

3. For example, Cho, in a videotape sent to NBC News, likened himself to Jesus Christ and Moses, saying his death would inspire countless generations (ABC News, 2007).

4. In January 2009, Haiyang Zhu, a male graduate student at VT, expressed romantic interest in Xin Yang, a female graduate student, who gently rebuffed him because she was engaged. Zhu reacted by pulling out a knife in a public café and decapitating her. The casualty toll was limited, and this would fall under the category of a domestic incident, but the brutality and lack of cause left a deep impression (Associated Press, 2009).

5. For official discussion of this event, see the 300-page report of the Virginia Tech Review Panel (2007).

6. Based on his own writings, in which he makes harsh comments about mothers and fathers, Cho may have hated his own parents. In a badly written but revealing play, *Richard McBeef*, Cho takes joy in falsely accusing his father of pedophilia, in causing physical clashes between his parents, and in framing his father for his (Cho's) accidental death (see Mackey, 2007). In addition, in a short story, he is highly critical of a cafeteria lady named Mrs. Vile (his mother worked in a cafeteria), who had the temerity to serve him a baloney sandwich rather than a more expensive lunch meat (Cho, 2006). In the end, Cho's antipathy seems directed at his parents for achieving modest rather than great financial success in food service and dry cleaning. However, his father, mother, and sister seem to be kind and loving people, who improved their own lives and tried to assist Cho.

7. One teacher in the English department recommended that Cho be removed from class because he was very disruptive: He took surreptitious pictures of young women's legs; he refused to participate in a class that was based on participation; and he sent an e-mail to all of his classmates damning them to hell because there had been a discussion in class about exotic food (such as eating escargot), and Cho had decided that this constituted an unforgiveable crime. Students were beginning to absent themselves because of Cho's presence. When Cho was withdrawn from this class, a second teacher took him on as an independent study student so that he could meet his requirements. Commentators in the aftermath of 4/16 found the first teacher too harsh and the latter too lenient; in reality they were only trying to help students. For an example of criticism directed at the English department, see Schlafly (2007).

8. Rev. Dong Cheol Lee, pastor of the One Mind Church, opined in an interview that "devil powers" afflicted Cho and that he had a personality that made him vulnerable to demonic forces. Michael Savage, in his radio program, the "Savage Nation," a few days after 4/16, citing the Ismael Ax moniker used in the packet sent to NBC News, argued that Cho was a Muslim and a supporter of Al-Qaeda. An extended treatise mailed to VT and found in the 4/16 archive claims that Cho was influenced negatively by Catholicism. Finally, Cho's mother said that she had been encouraged to consult a minister who had had success with troubled youth. She attended the church on and off for several months, but she decided against asking for assistance (Virginia Tech Review Panel, 2007).

9. The VT community did not engage in anti-Asian activity in the wake of events of 4/16. The community understood that the acts of 4/16 were produced by one individual and were not attributable to a race.

10. There were many reports of students at VT who tried to befriend Cho, and desisted only due to his inability to return friendship or even civility. See, by way of illustration, Duffy (2007).

11. At Lanza's home in Newtown, police found many weapons: nine knives, three Samurai swords, two rifles, 1,600 rounds of ammunition, and a spear. Lanza fired 154 bullets in the elementary school, using a Bushmaster .223 rifle and a Glock 10-mm handgun. Lanza used multiple magazines with 30-round capacity. See "Investigators" (2013).

12. Lanza had difficulty in German, but his grades overall were good (a 3.26 in seven classes carried to completion over four terms, from the summer of 2008 through the summer of 2009). Lanza refused to identify his gender and would not offer any comments on himself (Goldstein, 2013).

13. The most important document is Rodger's autobiography, "My Twisted World: The Story of Elliot Rodger" (2014b). One can review his last video, announcing his "Day of Retribution" (Rodger, 2014c). Between moments of deep self-pity and seething anger, with an occasional sneering laugh thrown in, a generally soft-spoken Rodger talks about wanting to create "mountains of skulls and rivers of blood." Rodger refers to himself as becoming God, and to others as becoming animals.

14. In Loughner's final days at Pima Community College, an instructor told him he would receive only partial credit because his assignment had been turned in late. Loughner claimed that the reduction of the grade interfered with his free speech rights, and police had to be called. See Reston, Rong-Gong, and Quinones (2011).

15. School officials and neighbors in Quick's middle-class neighborhood described Quick as friendly, but withdrawn. Quick's grandmother also expressed surprise. The latter said that Dylan was close to family, particularly his mother and father. However, the 85-year-old grandmother lived in Michigan and communicated with her grandson only over the telephone from time to time. See Plushnick-Masti and Lozano (2013).

16. See, for example, CNN Library (2014). Three of these took place at universities or colleges. There are many other lists that one could peruse as well, including those involving workplaces.

17. See "Clery Center" (n.d.).

18. All the Clery data reported here were extracted by using the Campus Safety and Security Data Analysis Cutting Tool (consultable at ope.ed.gov/security/).

19. I have not provided the data, due to lack of time and space. However, the material is available on request.

20. It discusses the case of Jackson Peebles, who had fought not to be required to take leave from his university to focus on suicidal concerns. He returned to his studies and committed suicide. On his life, see Cantero (2013).

References

ABC News. (2007, April 19). *Killer mails letter, photos, video to NBC*. Retrieved from http://abcnews.go.com/GMA/story?id=3055889

Abcarian, R., Garrison, J., & Groves, M. (2013, June 10). Santa Monica shooter's background steeped in trauma, violence. *Los Angeles Times*. Retrieved from http://articles.latimes.com/2013/jun/10/local/la-me-0611-santa-monica-shooting-20130611

Abdulsalam al-Zahrani, grad student admits to killing Binghamton University professor Richard Anton. (2011, May 20). *Huffington Post*. Retrieved from http://www.huffingtonpost.com/2011/05/20/abdulsalam-alzahrani-grad_n_864929.html

Adams, D. (2007, April 28). Seung Hui Cho: 'There was something evil aiding him.' *Roanoke Times*. Retrieved from http://www.roanoke.com/webmin/virginia_tech/seung-hui-cho-there-was-something-evil-aiding-him/article_b81a1174-7d98-5c92-8a67-aa8ebea21e3e.html

Arrest made in Temple student murder. (2013, January 4). Retrieved from http://6abc.com/archive/8941711

Associated Press. (2007, April 26). Memorial stone for gunman reappears. *Washington Post*. Retrieved from http://www.washingtonpost.com/wp-dyn/content/article/2007/04/25/AR2007042502110_pf.html

Associated Press. (2009, December 21). *Man pleads guilty in Va. Tech decapitation*. Retrieved from http://www.Nbcnews.com /id/34510604/ns/us_news-crime_and_courts/t/man-pleads-guilty-va-tech-decapitation/#.U8HPH1Ig-zc

Associated Press. (2012a, September 11). Ex-professor Amy Bishop pleads guilty to killing Alabama colleagues. *New York Daily News*. Retrieved from http://www.nydailynews.com/news/national/ex-professor-amy-bishop-pleads-guilty-killing-alabama-colleagues-article-1.1157187

Associated Press. (2012b, December 17). Adam Lanza took Western Connecticut State University courses when he was 16. *Huffington Post.* Retrieved from http://www.huffingtonpost.com/2012/12/17/adam-lanza-college-courses_n_2315431.html

Associated Press. (2013a, January 7). Suspect in killings deemed unfit. *New York Times.* Retrieved from http://www.nytimes.com/2013/01/08/us/suspect-in-oikos-university-killings-deemed-not-fit-for-trial.html?_r=0

Associated Press. (2013b, April 10). Neil A. MacInnis, Virginia mall shooting suspect, legally purchased shotgun: Police. *Huffington Post.* Retrieved from http://www.huffingtonpost.com/2013/04/16/neil-macinnis-legally-purchased-shotgun_n_3090972.html

Associated Press. (2014, June 11). *Prosecutor says Seattle campus shooter stopped taking his medication.* Retrieved from http://www.foxnews.com/us/2014/06/11/prosecutor-says-seattle-campus-shooter-stopped-taking-his-medication

Atkins, A. (2013, April 26). Right place, right time, right man for the job. *News Messenger.* Retrieved from http://ourvalley.org/right-place-right-time-right-man-for-the-job

Baker, A. (2010, September). Pace University student fatally shot in a robbery attempt. *New York Times.* Retrieved from http://www.nytimes.com/2010/09/30/nyregion/30pace.html?_r=0

Baker, M. (2014, July 10). SPU shooting suspect once had AK-47, 7 other firearms at home. *Seattle Times.* Retrieved from http://seattletimes.com/html/localnews/2024041234_spushootinggunsxml.html

Bamforth, A. (2014, June 7). Police: SPU shooter struggled with mental health problems, wanted to "to kill as many people as possible before killing himself." Retrieved from http://benswann.com/police-spu-shooter-struggled-with-mental-health-problems-wanted-to-to-kill-as-many-people-as-possible-before-killing-himself

Barakat, M. (2011, March 28). Jason M. Hamilton pleads guilty in Northern Virginia Community College shooting. *Huffington Post.* Retrieved from http://www.huffingtonpost.com/2011/03/28/jason-m-hamilton-pleads-g_n_841522.html

Bart, S. (2014). *"From where does the saying 'Save a life, save a whole world' originate?"* Retrieved from http://www.askmoses.com/en/article/192,2230417/From-where-does-the-saying-Save-a-life-save-a-whole-world-originate.html

Billeaud, J., & Tang, T. (2011, May 20). Jared Loughner at Pima Community College: Emails document an unstable personality. *Huffington Post.* Retrieved from http://www.huffingtonpost.com/2011/05/20/jared-loughner-at-pima-co_n_864548.html

Brown, E. (2013, June 11). Mother of Santa Monica College shooter John Zawahri expresses "great sadness" over shooting. *International Business Times.* Retrieved from http://www.ibtimes.com/mother-santa-monica-college-shooter-john-zawahri-expresses-great-sadness-over-shooting-1300321

Canadian Press. (2014, May 22). Matthew de Grood found fit to stand trial for allegedly killing five young people in Calgary's worst mass stabbing. *National Post.* Retrieved from http://news.nationalpost.com/news/canada/matthew-de-grood-found-fit-to-stand-trial-for-allegedly-killing-five-young-people-in-calgarys-worst-mass-stabbing

Cantero, C. (2013, December 29). Jackson Peebles, 21, had a habit of questioning authority and a 'deep desire to help humanity.' *Michigan Live*. Retrieved from http://www.mlive.com/news/kalamazoo/index.ssf/2013/12/kalamazoo_community_remembers_1.html

Caulfield, P. (2011, December 11). Friend of Virginia Tech shooter Ross Ashley says two went to gun range. *New York Daily News*. Retrieved from http://www.nydailynews.com/news/national/friend-virginia-tech-shooter-ross-ashley-gun-range-article-1.990007

Chapman, M. (2014, January 30). *Sandy Hook killer had 'movie depicting a man/boy relationship' on his PC*. Retrieved from http://www.cnsnews.com/news/article/michael-w-chapman/sandy-hook-killer-had-movie-depicting-manboy-relationship-his-pc

Cho, S.-H. (2006, September 20) *Baloney girl*, unpublished story in 4/16 archive.

Clery Center for Security on Campus. (n.d.). *Summary of the Jeanne Clery Act*. Retrieved from http://clerycenter.org/summary-jeanne-clery-act

Cloud, J. (2011, January 15). The troubled life of Jared Loughner. *Time*. Retrieved from http://content.time.com/time/magazine/article/0,9171,2042358,00.html

CNN Library. (2014, September 2). *25 deadliest mass shootings in the U.S.* Retrieved from http://www.cnn.com/2013/09/16/us/20-deadliest-mass-shootings-in-u-s-history-fast-facts

CNN Wire Staff. (2010, October 2). *University of Texas shooter was quiet, smart*. Retrieved from http://www.cnn.com/2010/CRIME/09/29/texas.university.shooting

Coffman, K. (2012, August 21). James Holmes, accused Colorado gunman, saw 3 mental health experts prior to deadly shooting. *Huffington Post*. Retrieved from http://www.huffingtonpost.com/2012/08/21/james-holmes-mental-health-colorado_n_1820450.html

Collection: Jared Lee Loughner. (n.d.). *Arizona Daily Star*. Retrieved from http://tucson.com/collection-jared-loughner/collection_808a756a-9645-11e2-9ef7-0019bb2963f4.html

Colby, E. B., Hamacher, B., & Finch, J. (2013, March 18). Student who killed himself at University of Central Florida had planned attack: Official. Retrieved from http://www.nbcmiami.com/news/Suspicious-Death-Investigated-at-University-of-Central-Florida-198750031.html.

Collins, T. (2012, April 3). One L. Goh, Oikos University shooting suspect, was upset about being teased over poor English skills: Police. *Huffington Post*. Retrieved from http://www.huffingtonpost.com/2012/04/03/one-l-goh-oikos-university-shooting-suspect_n_1399256.html

Conviction for local death row inmate John Thuesen affirmed. (2014, February 26). Retrieved from http://www.kbtx.com/home/headlines/Conviction-for-Local-Death-Row-Inmate-John-Thuesen-Affirmed-in-Brazos-County-247425141.html

Daily Mail Reporter. (2010, September 29). Terror on campus: Students dive for cover as gunman carrying AK47 opens fire in library of University of Texas. *Daily Mail*. Retrieved from http://www.dailymail.co.uk/news/article-1315903/University-Texas-shooting-Gunman-Colton-Tooley-opens-library.html

Davis, R. (2013, March 20). *UCF gunman, James Seevakumaran was a 'loner.'* Retrieved from http://www.mynews13.com/content/news/cfnews13/news/article .html/content/news/articles/cfn/2013/3/19/ucf_gunman_s_family_.html

Delaney, A. (2012, July 27). *James Holmes: Was the alleged shooter collecting unemployment insurance? Huffington Post.* Retrieved from http://www.huffingtonpost .com/2012/07/27/james-holmes-unemployment-insurance_n_1707367.html

Department of Emergency Services and Public Protection. (2013). *Sandy Hook Elementary School shooting reports.* Retrieved from http://cspsandyhookreport.ct.gov

Dick, D. (2011, February 8). YSU students describe post-shooting campus as 'dim.' *Vindicator.* Retrieved from http://www.vindy.com/news/2011/feb/08/angst-anger-sorrow/

Duffy, M. (2007, April 17). Inside Cho Seung-Hui's dorm. *Time.* Retrieved from www.time.com/time/nation/article/0,8599,161154800.html

Dujardin, P. (2009, November 11). Former student gets 14 years in shootings. *Daily Press.* Retrieved from http://articles.dailypress.com/2009-11-11/news/ 0911100086_1_maye-mental-illnesses-shooting

Farberov, S., & Golgowski, N. (2012, October 25). I gave him the nose job he always wanted: Woman 'shot lawyer boyfriend twice in the head . . . then four more times to stop the twitching.' *Daily Mail.* Retrieved from http://www.dailymail.co.uk/ news/article-2223787/Shayna-Hubers-Woman-shot-dead-lawyer-boyfriend-Ryan-Poston-giving-nose-job-wanted.html

Female escort, 19, charged in suffocation death of client. (2014, April 4). Retrieved from http://www.cbsnews.com/news/female-escort-19-charged-in-suffocation-death-of-client

Ferner, M. (2013, September 9). Secret James Holmes mental health report completed, given to court. *Huffington Post.* Retrieved from http://www.huffingtonpost .com/2013/09/09/secret-james-holmes-mental-report_n_3895534.html

Finnegan, L. (2010, September 30). Colton Tooley, UT shooter, had history of interest in gun control policy. *Huffington Post.* Retrieved from http://www.huffingtonpost .com/2010/09/30/colton-tooley-ut-shooter-_n_745292.html

Ferraro, R., & McHugh, B. (2010). Violence in the shadow of the ivory tower: Murder at the university. In Hemphill & Hephner LaBanc (Eds.). *Enough is enough* (pp. 1–38). Sterling, VA: Stylus.

Flegenheimer, M. (2013, December 27). Final report on Sandy Hook killings sheds new light on gunman's isolation. *New York Times.* Retrieved from http://www .nytimes.com/2013/12/28/nyregion/with-release-of-final-sandy-hook-shooting-report-investigation-is-said-to-be-over.html?pagewant

Follman, M. (2013, June 11). Santa Monica killer John Zawahri: A familiar profile. *Mother Jones.* Retrieved from http://www.motherjones.com/mojo/2013/06/santa-monica-john-zawahri-assault-rifle-high-capacity-magazines

Fox, L. (2013, November 25). Report: Sandy Hook shooter Adam Lanza was obsessed with mass shootings. *U.S. News World Report.* Retrieved from http://www.usnews .com/news/articles/2013/11/25/report-sandy-hook-shooter-adam-lanza-was-obsessed-with-mass-shootings

Gafni, M., Peele, T., Melvin, J., & Krupnick, M. (2012, April 3). Oakland university shooting: Accused Oikos University shooter One Goh was 'troubled,' 'angry,' said those who knew him. *Oakland Tribune.* Retrieved from http://www.insidebayarea

.com/top-stories/ci_20314383/oakland-school-rampage-suspect-sought-revenge
-against-administrator

Gibb, T. (2003, February 25). Shooter in 1996 Penn State killing recounts her past. *Post-Gazette*. Retrieved from http://old.post-gazette.com/localnews /20030225sniper0225p3.asp

Goldstein, S. (2011, November 4). Man gets life for fatally stabbing Dallas art institute student. *Dallas Morning News*. Retrieved from http://www.dallasnews .com/news/crime/headlines/20111104-man-gets-life-for-fatally-stabbing-dallas-art-institute-student.ece

Goldstein, S. (2013, April 2). Adam Lanza college records: Newtown shooter's bizarre questionnaire answers, good grades and creepy ID photo paint shocking portrait. *New York Daily News*. Retrieved from http://www.nydailynews.com/news/ national/lanza-college-records-suggest-troubling-state-mind-article-1.1305968

Gorman, R. (2014, January 11). Popular sorority member 'shot dead by another woman in front of terrified friends in road rage dispute.' *Daily Mail*. Retrieved from http://www.dailymail.co.uk/news/article-2537689/Woman-shot-dead-college-student-terrified-friend-road-rage-dispute.html

Grasgreen, A. (2014, January 2). Who protects the suicidal? *Inside Higher Education*. Retrieved from http://www.insidehighered.com/news/2014/01/02/suicide-ocr-again-tells-colleges-not-remove-self-threatening-students#sthash.Y2kpZm1h .dpbs

Griffin, A. (2013, December 28). Lanza's psychiatric treatment revealed in documents. *Hartford Courant*. Retrieved from http://articles.courant.com/2013-12-28/news/hc-lanza-sandy-hook-report1228-20131227_1_peter-lanza-adam-lanza-nancy-lanza

Gruver, M. (2012, December 2). Christopher Krumm attacked father James Krumm with bow and arrow, stabbed Heidi Arnold. *Huffington Post*. Retrieved from http://www.huffingtonpost.com/2012/12/02/christopher-krumm-james-heidi -arnold-attack-bow-and-arrow_n_2227151.html

Guarino, M. (2011, December 12). Virginia Tech shooting: Who was gunman Ross Truett Ashley? *Christian Science Monitor*. Retrieved from http://www.csmonitor. com/USA/2011/1212/Virginia-Tech-shooting-Who-was-gunman-Ross-Truett-Ashley

Herman, H. (2010, September 24). Oley man sentenced in slaying of ex-girlfriend at Gettysburg College. *Reading Eagle*. Retrieved from http://www2.readingeagle .com/article.aspx?id=251474

In memory of our fellow gauchos. (2014, May 29). *Daily Nexus*. Retrieved from http://dailynexus.com/2014-05-29/in-memory-of-our-fellow-gauchos

Ingold, J. (2013, April 4). Aurora theater shooting documents: Doctor reported James Holmes was threat to public. *Denver Post*. Retrieved from http://www .denverpost.com/ci_22955988/judge-unseals-warrants-affidavit-aurora-theater-shooting-case

Investigators: Adam Lanza surrounded by weapons at home; attack took less than 5 minutes. (2013, March 28). Retrieved from http://investigations.nbcnews .com/_news/2013/03/28/17501282-investigators-adam-lanza-surrounded-by -weapons-at-home-attack-took-less-than-5-minutes

James, S. D. (2010, February 19). *Shooter Amy Bishop likely schizophrenic says lawyer.* Retrieved from http://abcnews.go.com/Health/MindMoodNews/amy-bishop -lawyer-plead-insanity-alleged-university-alabama-shooter-schizophrenic/ story?id=9880257

James Seevakumaran, evicted UCF student, ID'd as man found shot dead on campus; planned wider attack, police say. (2013, March 18). Retrieved from http:// www.cbsnews.com/news/james-seevakumaran-evicted-ucf-student-idd-as-man-found-shot-dead-on-campus-planned-wider-attack-police-say

Jared Loughner had 5 run-ins with college police. (2011, January 10). Retrieved from http://www.cbsnews.com/news/jared-loughner-had-5-run-ins-with-college-police

Jared Loughner to be forced to take anti-psychotic medication. (2011, July 27). Retrieved from http://www.cnn.com/2011/CRIME/07/27/arizona.loughner.medication

Jason Hamilton pleads guilty to NVCC Woodbridge shooting. (2011, March 28). Retrieved from http://www.tbd.com/articles/2011/03/jason-hamilton-pleads -guilty-to-nvcc-woodbridge-shooting-57388.html

Jennings, D. (2010, April 2). UTD student pleads guilty to stabbing teaching assistant. *Dallas Morning News.* Retrieved from http://www.dallasnews.com/ news/crime/headlines/20100401-UTD-student-pleads-guilty-to-stabbing-2529 .ece

Jones, G. (2012, June 10). *Media missed horrific, tragic crime.* WBRC Fox 6. Retrieved from http://www.myfoxal.com/story/17859473/commentary-trayvon-vs -christian-newsom

Jonsson, P. (2014, June 7). Seattle Pacific shooting: Despite 'rage inside,' Aaron Ybarra found 'not detainable.' *Christian Science Monitor.* Retrieved from http://www .csmonitor.com/USA/2014/0607/Seattle-Pacific-shooting-Despite-rage-inside-Aaron-Ybarra-found-not-detainable-video

Kang, J. C. (2013, March 28). That other school shooting. *New York Times.* Retrieved from http://www.nytimes.com/2013/03/31/magazine/should-it-matter-that-the-shooter-at-oikos-university-was-korean.html?pagewanted=all&_r=0

Keefe, P. R. (2013, February 11). A loaded gun: A mass shooter's tragic past. *New Yorker.* Retrieved from http://www.newyorker.com/reporting/2013/02/11/130211fa_fact_keefe?currentPage=all

Kemp, J., Hutchinson, B., & Cunningham, J. (2013, January 1). Suspect in fatal stabbing had been stalking ill-fated ex-girlfriend. for months after she ended relationship: Victim's brother. *New York Daily News.* Retrieved from http://www .nydailynews.com/new-york/uptown/suspect-stabbing-death-allegedly-stalked -victim-article-1.1231244

Kennedy, H. (2011, January 10). Gabrielle Giffords shooting: Brave bystanders help subdue Arizona killer Jared Lee Loughner. *Daily News.* Retrieved from http://www.nydailynews.com/news/national/gabrielle-giffords-shooting-brave-bystanders-subdue-arizona-killer-jared-lee-loughner-article-1.1491

Kimzey, K. (2013, June 10). *Man sentenced to 30 years in killing of transgender college student.* Retrieved from http://www.goupstate.com/article/20130610/ ARTICLES/306101012

Korfage, S. (2014, February 14). Quentin Truehill murder trial: Medical examiner says Vincent Binder tried to defend himself. *Florida Times-Union.* Retrieved from

http://jacksonville.com/news/crime/2014-02-14/story/quentin-truehill-murder
-trial-medical-examiner-says-vincent-binder-tried

Lacey, M. (2011, May 25). Suspect in shooting of Giffords ruled unfit for trial. *New York Times*. Retrieved from http://www.nytimes.com/2011/05/26/us/26loughner
.html?pagewanted=all&_r=0

Launer, D. (2014, July 9). How I tried to help Elliot Rodger. *BBC News Magazine*. Retrieved from http://www.bbc.com/news/magazine-28197785

Lavergne, G. (1997). *A sniper in the tower*. Denton: University of North Texas Press.

Leahy, E. (2013, September 18). *Guns do not make a nation safer, say doctors in a new study*. Retrieved from http://www.elsevier.com/connect/guns-do-not-make-a-nation-safer-say-doctors-in-new-study

Lee, J. (2007, April 19). *Real paranoia: Was Seung-Hui Cho a mind-controlled assassin?* Retrieved from www.freedom-center.org/seung-hui-cho-was-mind
-controlled-assassin

Lewis, B., & Sampson, Z. C. (2011, December 9). Ross Truett Ashley, Virginia Tech shooter, was 22-year-old Radford University student. *Huffington Post*. Retrieved from http://www.huffingtonpost.com/2011/12/09/ross-truett-ashley-radford-university-student_n_1140247.html

Little, R. (2012, April 25). Man confesses to killing 2 Polk State students, police say. *Ledger*. Retrieved from http://www.theledger.com/article/20120425/NEWS
/120429559

Lozano, J. (2013, April 11). *Warrant: Texas suspect interested in cannibalism*. Retrieved from http://bigstory.ap.org/article/texas-college-knife-attack-suspect
-be-court

Lutz, A. (2012, July 25). How James Holmes went from shy nerd to accused cold-blooded killer. *Business Insider*. Retrieved from http://www.businessinsider.com/
james-holmes-biography-2012-7

Lysiak, M. (2013). *Newtown, an American tragedy*. New York, NY: Gallery Books.

Mackey, B. (2007, April 22). *The annotated Richard McBeef*. Retrieved from http://
www.somethingawful.com/news/richard-mcbeef/1

Martinez, M., & Carter, C. (2013, March 28). *New details: Loughner's parents took gun, disabled car to keep him home*. Retrieved from http://www.cnn
.com/2013/03/27/justice/arizona-loughner-details

McLaughlin, M. (2012, August 27). James Holmes asked about dysphoric mania, sent 'bad news' message before Aurora shooting. *Huffington Post*. Retrieved from http://www.huffingtonpost.com/2012/08/27/james-holmes-dysphoric-mania
-aurora-shooting_n_1833228.html

Morava, K. (2013, May 11). Defendant's own words describe killing of college student near Asher. *Shawnee News-Star*. Retrieved from http://www.news-star.com/
article/20130510/News/130519956

Nano, S. (2012, December 15). No link between Asperger's syndrome and violence say experts. *Huffington Post*. Retrieved from http://www.huffingtonpost
.com/2012/12/16/violence-aspergers-syndrome-adam-lanza--newtown-
shooting_n_2312545.html

Nelson, S. (2013, April 10). Texas stabber Dylan Andrew Quick was bullied, fantasized about murdering with knife, reports say. *U.S. News & World Report*. Retrieved from http://www.usnews. com/news/newsgram/ articles/ 2013/04/10/

texas-stabber-dylan-andrew-quick-was-bullied-fantasized-about-murdering-with-knife-reports-say

Nye, J. (2014, March 10). 'I wish he had never been born': Adam Lanza's father breaks his silence on 'evil' son who killed 20 children at Sandy Hook school in first interview since tragedy. *Daily Mail*. Retrieved from http://www.dailymail.co.uk/news/article-2577174/I-wish-never-born-Adam-Lanzas-father-makes-startling -admission-son-killed-20-children-Sandy-Hook-school-interview-tragedy.html

Parascandola, R., & Kemp, J. (2011, December 1). Ex-boyfriend of Rita Morelli, Italian college student murdered in E. Harlem, says he was under spell when he killed her. *New York Daily News*. Retrieved from http://www.nydailynews .com/news/crime/ex-boyfriend-rita-morelli-italian-college-student-murdered-e-harlem-spell-killed-article-1.985666

Plushnick-Masti, R., & Lozano, J. (2013). Dylan Quick charged in Lone Star stabbing rampage. *Huffington Post*. Retrieved from http://www.huffingtonpost.com /2013/04/10/dylan-quick-lone-star-college-stabbing_n_3050388. html

Powell, M. (2014, April 16). Videos at hearing give insight to mall shooter Mac-Innis. *Roanoke Times*. Retrieved from http://www.roanoke.com/news/crime/ christiansburg/teen-charged-in-community-college-shooting-set-to-plea-this/ article_bb5254f4-c55d-11e3-9eb2-001a4bcf6878.html

Report says school shooter Lanza had controversial sensory condition, Asperger's. (2013, February 21). Retrieved from http://www.foxnews.com/us/2013/02/21/ sandy-hook-shooter-lanza-reportedly-had-sensory-integration-disorder-asperger

Reston, M., Rong-Gong, L., & Quinones, S. (2011, January 12). Jared Loughner was no stranger to police. *Los Angeles Times*. Retrieved from http://articles .latimes.com/2011/jan/12/ nation/la-na-jared-loughner-20110113

Rodger, E. (2014a). Day of retribution [Video file]. *New York Times*. Retrieved from http://www.nytimes.com/video/us/100000002900707/youtube-video-retribution .html

Rodger, E. (2014b). My twisted world: The story of Elliot Rodger. Retrieved from http://www.ibtimes.com/read-elliot-rodgers-140-page-memoir-manifesto-he -wrote-prior-his-shooting-university-1589868

Sadowsky, J. (2013, May 31). UCF releases new photos from UCF gunman's room, computer: Seevakumaran manifesto. *Knight News*. Retrieved from http://knight news.com/2013/05/ucf-releases-new-photos-from-ucf-gunmans-room-computer -seevakumaran-manifesto

Saletan, W. (2011, January 11). Friendly firearms: Gabrielle Giffords and the perils of guns: How an armed hero nearly shot the wrong man. *Slate*. Retrieved from http://www.slate.com/articles/health_and_science/human_nature/2011/01/ friendly_firearms.html

Salinas, O. (2014, April 6). *New River Valley shooter pleads guilty to four felony charges*. Retrieved from http://www.wdbj7.com/news/local/new-river-valley-mall -shooting-suspect-due-in-court-tuesday-morning/25511176

Santana, S., & Nolin, R. (2009, May 30). 2 women shot dead at Chevron Station. *Sun Sentinel*. Retrieved from http://articles.sun-sentinel.com/2009-05-30/ news/0905290418_1_domestic-violence-police-station-all-night-gas-station

Schlafly, P. (2007, May 9). What Cho learned in the English department. *Eagle Forum*. Retrieved from http://www.eagleforum.org/column/2007/may07/07-05-09.html

Shaffer, C. (2014, February 18). *Cleveland man fatally stabbed in heart; woman charged with murder.* Retrieved from http://www.cleveland.com/metro/index.ssf/ 2014/02/cleveland_man_ fatally_ stabbed_1.html

Shannon, K. (2010, September 29). UT shooter Colton Tooley described as intelligent, unemotional. *Huffington Post.* Retrieved from http://www.huffingtonpost .com/2010/09/29/ut-shooter-colton-tooley-_0_n_744254. html

Shaw, A. (2013, April 13). *Weapons, ammo used in Va. community college attack may have been posted online by shooter.* Retrieved from http://abcnews.go.com/US/ neil-macinnis-online-posts-detail-weapons-ammo-va/story?id=18946729

Starviego. (2013, April 13). 4-12-13 New River Community College, Virginia. [Online forum comment]. Retrieved from http://signofthetimes.yuku.com/ topic/1509/ 41213-New-River-Community-College-Virginia

Steffen, J. (2013, December 1). Evidence details twisted path that led Austin Sigg to Jessica Ridgeway. *Denver Post.* Retrieved from http://www.denverpost.com/news/ ci_24631031/evidence-details-twisted-path-that-led-austin-sigg

Stevenson, C. (n.d.). *Gun violence strikes another Virginia school.* Retrieved from http://weapons.academic.wlu.edu/another-tragedy-hits-virginian-schools

Suspect kills self in Ohio State shooting, police say. (2010, March 9). Retrieved from http://www.cnn.com/ 2010/CRIME/03/09/ohio.state.shooting

Sussman, A. (2012, July 25). James Holmes, Aurora theater gunman, may have used federal student grants to fund shooting. *Huffington Post.* Retrieved from http://www.huffingtonpost.com/2012/07/25/james-holmes-nih-student-grants -shooting_n_1702740.html

Tuohy, L. (2014, June 27). Seth Mazzaglia found guilty in rape, murder of university student. *Huffington Post.* Retrieved from http://www.huffingtonpost .com/2014/06/27/seth-mazzaglia-guilty-rape-murder-unh_n_5537894.html

UCF gunman James Seevakumaran's roommate speaks. (2013, March 2). [Video file]. Retrieved from http://www.baynews9.com/content/news/baynews9/news/ article.html/content/news/ articles/cfn/ 2013/3/20/roommate_in_ucf_plot.html

Vann, D. (2009, February 12). Portrait of the school shooter as a young man. *Esquire.* Retrieved from http://www.esquire.com/features/steven-kazmierczak-0808

Vega, C., Gard, C., Vojtech, J., Keohane, E., & Berardi, T. (2014, May 30). Santa Barbara killer smiled before shooting, survivor says. *Good Morning America.* Retrieved from http://abcnews.go.com/US/santa-barbara-killer-elliotrodger-smil ed-shooting-survivor/story?id=23923970

Virginia Tech Review Panel. (2007, April 16). *Mass shootings at Virginia Tech: Report of the Review Panel presented to Governor Kaine.* Retrieved May 26, 2015 from http://cdm16064.contentdm.oclc.org/cdm/ref/collection/p266901coll4/id/904

Wadman, M. (2010, May 12). Universities: Life after death. *Nature.* Retrieved May 28, 2015 from http://www.nature.com/news/2010/100512/full/465150a.html

Williams, R. (2007, June 21). No drugs found in Cho's body. *Roanoke Times.* Retrieved from http://www.roanoke.com/webmin/virginia_tech/no-drugs-found -in-cho-s-body/article_26ac1869-5720-56f1-8c7b-2df44165b1be.html

Wood, D. B. (2012, April 2). Oakland shooter's connections to religious university under scrutiny. *Christian Science Monitor.* Retrieved from http://www.csmonitor .com/USA/2012/0402/Oakland-shooter-s-connections-to-religious-university- under-scrutiny

Woods, J. (2010, September 30). At the U of Texas, a suicide mistaken for a school shooting. *Huffington Post*. Retrieved, from http://www.huffingtonpost.com/john -woods/at-the-university-of- texa_b_745390.html

Yu, X. (2011, September 30). Ex-Harvard student, Brittany Smith, sentenced to three years in prison. *Harvard Crimson*. Retrieved from http://www.thecrimson .com/article/2011/9/30/brittany-smith-harvard-shooting-sentenced

2 Concealed Carry Legislation and Changing Campus Policies

Kerry Brian Melear and Mark St. Louis

GUN CONTROL legislation affecting higher education has been enacted across the country and across a range of alternative postures in the wake of campus tragedies during recent years, and the issue is polarizing indeed. In a 2013 survey of approximately 400 college presidents, 95% of presidents did not support concealed weapons on college campuses, noting that recent campus shootings and "pressure from pro firearm groups (e.g., National Rifle Association) have led to political pressures to permit concealed carry of firearms on college campuses" (Price et al., 2014, p. 3). Similarly, approximately 80% of students surveyed at a number of Midwestern universities opposed concealed weapons on campus (Doubleday, 2013). This position directly opposed the pro-gun advocacy group Students for Concealed Carry on Campus (SCCC), which recently sued The Ohio State University, arguing that its ban on guns was overbroad (Drabold, 2014). SCCC is a nonpartisan organization composed of 43,000 college students, professors, parents, and others "who believe that holders of state-issued concealed handgun licenses should be allowed the same measure of personal protection on college campuses that current laws afford them virtually everywhere else" (Students for Concealed Carry on Campus, n.d.). The political tensions abiding between these two philosophies are not likely to be bridged any time soon and have been drivers of legislative activity on both sides.

The Second Amendment has long played a central role in debates concerning gun control; state laws shape the contours of higher education policy and practice in this regard. This chapter briefly outlines the Second Amendment and related key U.S. Supreme Court decisions, and then surveys state firearm laws that resonate within higher education. State laws permitting concealed weapons on campus are discussed, notable recent legislation is identified, and litigation that surrounds institutional policies and state laws affecting higher education are explored.

The Second Amendment and the U.S. Supreme Court

The Second Amendment to the U.S. Constitution provides that "a well regulated Militia, being necessary to the security of a free State, the right of the people to keep and bear Arms, shall not be infringed" (U.S. Constitution, Second Amendment, 1791). The language of the amendment has long generated discussion and debate regarding whether it may apply collectively or individually to citizens.

In 2008, the U.S. Supreme Court rendered a decision in *District of Columbia v. Heller* that settled the question, narrowly ruling that the Second Amendment protects the individual's right to possess firearms to be used for a lawful purpose, such as self-defense (*District of Columbia v. Heller*, 2008; Hatt, 2011). In *District of Columbia v. Heller*, the Supreme Court struck down a District of Columbia law prohibiting the possession of firearms, concluding that the Second Amendment guarantees "the individual right to possess and carry weapons in case of confrontation" (*District of Columbia v. Heller*, 2008). The ruling upset the court's previously long-held posture disfavoring an individual application of the Second Amendment, articulated in *United States v. Miller* (1939), in which the court concluded that the purpose of the Second Amendment related to the militia. In 2010, the Court revisited the Second Amendment and buttressed its individual applicability, holding in *McDonald v. City of Chicago* that a ban on handguns in Chicago was unconstitutional because the right to keep and bear arms is protected by the Second Amendment, which applies to the states by incorporation through the due process clause of the Fourteenth Amendment, underscoring the decision in *District of Columbia v. Heller*.

State Laws and Higher Education

State legislation concerning firearms on campus varies widely according to the carriage and demeanor of a particular region, and as

LaPoint (2010) noted, "It is clear that both sides in the debate over concealed carry on college campuses have strong convictions, with neither side willing to concede" (p. 19). Although the majority of colleges and universities prohibit guns on campus, federal law provides no guidance in regard to such prohibitions, leaving the issue to the states, which are divided on the matter (Skorton & Altschuler, 2013).

In the wake of college campus tragedies, as well as the 2012 shootings at Sandy Hook Elementary School, in which 26 students and staff were killed (Flegenheimer, 2013), state legislative activity concerning firearms on college campuses has been robust. According to the National Conference of State Legislatures (2014), there are currently 21 states that ban concealed weapons on college campuses,[1] and in 22 states the decision of whether to permit or allow concealed weapons is reached individually by the college, university, or governing system.[2]

Legislation Permitting Concealed Carry on the College Campus

Seven states have passed laws specifically providing for concealed carry permits on college campuses (National Conference of State Legislatures, 2014).[3] Of these, Utah is the only state to specifically identify publicly funded colleges and universities as governmental entities lacking the authority to ban concealed carry permits on their premises, and, as a result, all 10 institutions allow concealed carry on their campuses ("National Conference of State Legislatures," 2014; Utah Code, § 53-5a-102, 2013).

In Wisconsin, although a concealed carry permit is required, colleges and universities may prohibit it by clearly and prominently posting signage at all entrances to a building (National Conference of State Legislatures, 2014; Wis. Stat. § 991.11.82.2a, 2011). Similarly, in Kansas, concealed firearms are not prohibited on college campuses; however, Kansas law permits institutions to prohibit concealed carry in buildings considered appropriately secure by clearly posting signage stating this prohibition (Kan. Stat. Ann. § 75-7c10, 2012; National Conference of State Legislatures, 2014). Governing boards may apply for exemptions every 4 years (Kan. Stat. Ann. § 75-7c10, 2012; National Conference of State Legislatures, 2014). In Mississippi, a 2011 law holds that a person who is licensed to carry a concealed weapon and "voluntarily complete[s] an instructional course in the safe handling and use of firearms offered by an instructor certified by a nationally recognized organization. . . , or by any other organization approved by the Department of Public Safety," may carry a concealed weapon on a college or university campus (Miss. Code Ann. § 97-37-1, 2011; National Conference of State Legislatures, 2014).

Idaho is the most recent state to pass legislation allowing concealed weapons on college campuses. Although the Idaho legislature had wholly occupied the field of firearms regulation within the state, it had permitted public colleges and universities to set their own policies regarding firearms on campuses. That changed on July 1, 2014, when Senate Bill 1254 became law in Idaho. Somewhat confusingly, although the bill acknowledged that the board of regents of the University of Idaho and the boards of trustees of the state colleges and universities have the authority to create rules and regulations "relating to firearms," the bill significantly limited the scope of that authority by refusing to extend it to "regulating or prohibiting the otherwise lawful possession, carrying or transporting of firearms or ammunition by persons licensed under section 18-3302H or 18-3302K, Idaho Code" (Senate Bill 1254 § 4, 18-33-9[2], 2013–2014).

The constitutional argument raised against this bill is quite interesting, albeit fairly narrow. The University of Idaho actually predates Idaho's admission to the union as a state, and Idaho's constitution specifically granted the University of Idaho the power to administer its day-to-day affairs. Therefore, blanket legislative acts, unless they actually amend the state constitution, that encroach on the constitutional authority of the University of Idaho to administer the university are unconstitutional (DeSantis, 2014). For example, in 1921 the Idaho Supreme Court held that legislation requiring the university to turn over funds from the sale of its property to the state was unconstitutional because the university had the right to control its own funds (*State ex rel. Black v. State Board of Education*, 1921). Whether a similar challenge would succeed against Senate Bill 1254 remains to be seen. Regardless, such a potential challenge would apply only to the University of Idaho and would seem to have no effect on other public colleges and universities in Idaho.

Though all eight presidents of Idaho's public colleges and universities fought against this legislation, Idaho universities began preparing their campuses for compliance within weeks of the governor signing the bill (Russell, 2014). Boise State University, for example, began revising policies and procedures to clarify what would change when the new law took effect and what would remain the same. Individuals with proper licenses would be allowed to carry concealed weapons on campus, except in residence halls and entertainment venues, whereas open carried weapons would remain banned everywhere on campus (Boise State University, n.d.). Additionally, the university was clear that it would not alter its immediate response to reports of a gun on university property (Graf, 2014). Other institutions, such as Idaho State University, began arming campus law enforcement officers for the first time (Zuckerman, 2014).

Recent Legislative Activity of Note to Higher Education

The landscape of legislation related to concealed carry has shifted extensively in the past few years. Administrators in higher education will have to continue to watch the trends, state by state, and anticipate legislative trends that will impact their given campuses. Some of the more recent and interesting changes are detailed here as an introduction to trends and implications.

Alaska

In sweeping language, a 2013 measure was passed in Alaska prohibiting state and municipal agencies, specifically defining the University of Alaska as such an agency, from using assets to implement or aid in the implementation of any federal law that would infringe on an Alaskan's Second Amendment right to keep and bear arms (Chapter 52 SLA 13, 2013). This measure was introduced as part of a perceived movement toward express protection of Second Amendment rights (Parker, 2013). However, the law did not prohibit the University of Alaska from implementing regulations of its own, free of any federal law, limiting firearms possession on its campus. In fact, the university specifically prohibits the possession of firearms in "buildings or parts of buildings owned or controlled by the university," as well as at university sporting, entertainment, or educational events (University of Alaska, 2014, p. 2).

Arkansas

In Arkansas, a controversial bill was passed in 2013 that allows properly trained and licensed employees to carry concealed handguns on post-secondary campuses, provided the governing board does not adopt a policy prohibiting the activity (Arkansas Act No. 226, 2013). Any such policies expire after 1 year and must be annually readopted (Arkansas Act No. 226, 2013). This bill contains an opt-out provision, and every university in the state has chosen to do so ("Laws Taking Effect," 2013), garnering national attention during that process (Kingkade, 2013).

Texas

Texas legislation passed in 2013 relates to the transportation and storage of firearms or ammunition on private and public college and university campuses, but in the context of concealed carry permits (Tex. Bus. & Com. Code § 411.2032, 2013). According to this statute, institutions of higher education cannot adopt or enforce any measure that prohibits or restricts the storage or transportation of a firearm or ammunition in a locked, privately owned vehicle by any person (student or otherwise) who holds a valid concealed carry permit in Texas (Tex. Bus. & Com. Code § 411.2032, 2013).

New York

New York's state law—the Secure Ammunition and Firearms Enforcement (SAFE) Act, S2230 (2013)—was passed as a direct result of the Newtown tragedy and was perhaps the most publicly followed gun control legislation of 2013. Because it involves litigation, it is discussed later in this chapter.

Georgia

On July 1, 2014, two bills became law in Georgia: House Bill 826 and House Bill 60. Both bills modified the same section of the Official Code of Georgia Annotated, specifically section 16-11-127.1, which originally stated:

> A person who is licensed in accordance with Code Section 16-11-
> 129 or issued a permit pursuant to Code Section 43-38-10, [may
> possess a concealed firearm] when such person carries or picks up
> a student at a school building, school function, or school property
> or on a bus or other transportation furnished by the school or a per-
> son who is licensed in accordance with Code Section 16-11-129 or
> issued a permit pursuant to Code Section 43-38-10 when he or she
> has any weapon legally kept within a vehicle when such vehicle is
> parked at such school property or is in transit through a designated
> school zone. (Ga. Stat. Ann. § 16-11-127.1)

Confusingly, the amendments made to 16-11-127.1 by HB 826 and HB 60 conflict with one another.

HB 826 states that an individual "licensed in accordance with Code Section 16-11-129 or issued a permit pursuant to Code Section 43-38-10" may possess a concealed firearm "when he or she is within a school safety zone or on a bus or other transportation furnished by a school" (Ga. HB 826[c][6], 2013–2014). A *school safety zone* is defined as "any real property or building owned by or leased to any school or postsecondary institution" (Ga. HB 826[c] [6], 2013–2014). Therefore, HB 826 has been interpreted as allowing individuals who are licensed to carry concealed firearms to do so on college or university property, including within buildings.

HB 60, however, which has been dubbed the "Guns Everywhere Bill" in the national press, is ironically, in the context of college and university campuses, more limiting (Richinick, 2014). Whereas HB 826 specifies a broad authorization, HB 60 allows licensed individuals to possess a concealed firearm in a school safety zone *only* "when such person carries or picks up a student within a school safety zone" or is "in transit through a designated school safety zone" (Ga. HB 60 §1-6 [c][7], 2013–2014).

Some have argued that the two bills are, in fact, not in conflict. Rather, HB 60 and 826 both state that concealed firearms may be allowed in vehicles, but HB 826 goes further, expanding the areas where a concealed firearm may be permitted. As the vice president and legal counsel for Georgia Carry has stated, if you place all the word changes from both bills together "you end with a cogent paragraph that means something" (Campbell, 2014). Others, such as Georgia attorney general Sam Olens, disagree. In a memo titled "Frequently Asked Questions Regarding Weapons Law Amendments

Taking Effect on July 1, 2014," Attorney General Olens explained (a) the bills are in conflict with one another, and (b) although both bills took effect on July 1, House Bill 60 was signed by the governor on April 23, whereas House Bill 826 was signed on April 22, so "the provisions of House Bill 60 control" (Simms, 2014, para. 9). Therefore, Olens writes, there is a

> general prohibition against carrying weapons in a school safety zone (which includes the real property or buildings of public or private elementary schools, secondary schools, technical schools, vocational schools, colleges or universities); however, a person who possesses a weapons carry license may have a weapon when carrying or picking up a student and may have a weapon in a vehicle that is in transit or parked within a school safety zone. (Simms, 2014, para. 9)

It appears that public colleges and universities in Georgia have embraced Olen's interpretation, and, as a result, little has changed in Georgia in terms of campus firearms policies. At the University of Georgia–Athens, for example, the general rule remains that firearms are prohibited on campus unless there is an exception, such as "the possession of weapons or devices which are legal to possess within a motor vehicle" (Williamson, n.d., p. 2).

Litigation, Institutional Policies, and State Laws Affecting Higher Education

Recent litigation in Oregon, Colorado, and Florida successfully overturned longstanding campus bans on firearms. In New York, however, gun control legislation has survived legal proceedings in federal court. This section will briefly survey litigation and state laws affecting higher education, as well as associated institutional policy responses.

Oregon

In 2011, the Oregon Court of Appeals concluded that an Oregon State Board of Higher Education administrative rule that imposed sanctions on persons who possess or use firearms while on university property exceeded the scope of the agency's authority and was thus invalid (*Oregon Firearms v. Board of Higher Education*, 2011). The ruling stirred considerable controversy and was closely followed by academic and news media outlets (Grasgreen, 2011; Graves, 2011a; Keller, 2011). The appeals court's ruling elicited an administrative response: In 2012 the Oregon higher education board unanimously adopted a policy that banned guns from classrooms, buildings, residence halls, and sporting events, although the policy did not extend to holders of concealed carry permits (Graves, 2012). The Oregon University System ultimately elected not to appeal the ruling, and the system's chancellor indicated that other procedures were viable: "Instead [of appealing], we have started work on internal processes that are already in place or that we can put in place that will maintain a reasonable and satisfactory level of campus safety and security" (Graves, 2011b, para. 3).

Colorado

In *Regents of the University of Colorado v. Students for Concealed Carry on Campus* (2012), the Supreme Court of Colorado addressed whether the university's 1994 campus weapons ban violated the Colorado Concealed Carry Act (CCA) and the Colorado Constitution's right to bear arms. A student group that favors concealed carry permits brought the suit, which a Colorado district court dismissed. An appellate court reversed that decision, however, and the Supreme Court of Colorado affirmed that ruling, stating the following:

> [T]he CCA's comprehensive statewide purpose, broad language, and narrow exclusions show that the General Assembly intended to divest the Board of Regents of its authority to regulate concealed handgun possession on campus. Accordingly, we agree with the court of appeals that, by alleging the Policy violates the CCA, the Students have stated a claim for relief. (*Regents of the University of Colorado v. Students for Concealed Carry on Campus*, 2012, p. 497)

The decision led to unease among faculty and staff of Colorado colleges and universities, whereas gun rights proponents argued that they should not be denied the right to protect themselves (Frosch, 2012). In a statement underscoring the tension between concerned administrators and the court, the president of the University of Colorado noted his disagreement with the ruling:

We are disappointed the Colorado Supreme Court determined that
the Board of Regents does not, in this instance, have the constitutional and statutory authority to determine what policies will best
promote the health and welfare of the university's students, faculty, staff and visitors, whose safety is our top priority. The Board
of Regents is in the best position to determine how we meet that
imperative. (Grasgreen, 2012, para. 7)

Florida

Although there has not been a recent legislative change in Florida
regarding firearms on campuses, recent activity in the courts has
forced colleges and universities in the state to change their interpretation of existing state firearms laws. Colleges and universities
in Florida previously had blanket firearms prohibitions in place on
their campuses. Then, in December 2013, the 2nd District Court of
Appeals ruled in favor of Florida Carry, Inc., in its suit against the
University of North Florida (UNF).

Florida Carry sought to invalidate UNF's prohibition against
individuals keeping firearms inside personal vehicles located on
UNF's property. Florida Carry argued that although Florida Statute
790.115(2)(a) prohibited the possession of a firearm on school property unless part of a school-sponsored event, the legislature created
an exception through 790.25(5), which allows firearms to be kept in a
private conveyance as long as they are securely encased (*Florida Carry
Inc. v. University of North Florida,* 2013). UNF countered that Florida
Statute 790.115(2)(a)3 created an exception to this exception, in that
"school districts" could "adopt policies to waive the secure encase-
ment exception." UNF, therefore, argued that its regulation prohibiting firearms in vehicles was merely the university applying that waiver
(*Florida Carry Inc. v. University of North Florida,* 2013).

The 2nd District, however, agreed with Florida Carry that public
colleges and universities in the state of Florida, including UNF, are
not "school districts" and therefore could not exercise the waiver.
Because the legislature preempted the entire field of firearms regulation through Florida Statute 790.33(1), and because UNF lacked any
specific grant of legislative authority to independently regulate firearms on its campus, the court struck down UNF's firearms regulation.

Florida's public colleges and universities began updating their
regulations following this ruling. Some institutions amended their

regulations to expressly state that firearms are now permitted in private conveyances if secured. Others, such as the University of South Florida (USF), have preferred a more flexible approach, simply maintaining that firearms are prohibited on campus unless explicitly permitted. Florida Carry prefers the former. Although Florida Carry will continue pressuring schools to expressly state that firearms are allowed in personal vehicles, they do not intend to litigate against USF because its regulation "appears to be a good faith attempt to resolve the issue" (Hayes, 2014). Regardless, the 2nd District has reinforced that the legislature, and not individual institutions of higher education, will make decisions regarding where firearms are allowed and prohibited.

Additional challenges have also followed the December 2013 decision. For example, Florida Carry has filed suit against the University of Florida to overturn its regulation prohibiting the possession of firearms in on-campus student housing. Florida Carry has argued that (a) the university is preempted from regulating firearms on its campus, and (b) the prohibition against keeping a firearm in one's home is unconstitutional. At the time of writing, the University of Florida had submitted a motion to dismiss, for which no decision had yet been reached.

New York

Unlike in Oregon and Colorado, sweeping gun legislation that passed in New York largely survived its first legal test in federal court. As previously noted, in early 2013, the New York State Assembly passed the Secure Ammunition and Firearms Enforcement (SAFE) Act, S2230 (2013), which received bipartisan support and was signed into law just over 1 month after the tragic campus shootings at Sandy Hook Elementary School (Koplovitz, 2013). Included among its many provisions were a ban on the sale of assault weapons, a requirement directing mental health professionals to report patients believed to be a danger to themselves or others, a requirement for background checks related to the private sale of guns, and a ban on magazines holding more than seven rounds of ammunition (Koplovitz, 2013).

The law immediately stimulated litigation. In *New York State Rifle and Pistol Association v. Cuomo* (2013), gun owners, purveyors, and gun-rights advocacy groups challenged the law in federal court, arguing, among other claims, that its provisions violated the Second Amendment. A federal district court largely disagreed, however, and concluded that many of the major provisions of the law "further the state's important interest in public safety, and do not impermissibly infringe on Plaintiffs' Second Amendment rights" (*New York State Rifle and Pistol Association v. Cuomo*, 2013). The provision limiting magazines to seven rounds was stricken, and gun control advocates considered the ruling a victory (Law Center to Prevent Gun Violence, 2014).

Of course, a significant number of the firearms on college and university campuses are in the hands of campus or local officers. In fact, many departments possess armories that include surplus military equipment acquired under the Department of Defense's 1033 program. Between 2006 and April 2014 the Pentagon distributed 79,288 assault rifles, 11,959 bayonets, hundreds of helicopters, and even mine-resistant vehicles to police departments across the United States (Rezvani, Pupovac, Eads, & Fisher, 2014). Although only a portion of these arms have gone to campus police or local departments near campuses, more than 100 college campuses have participated in the 1033 program since last December (Grasgreen, 2014). For example, Florida International University's campus police received military-grade rifles, and The Ohio State University obtained a mine-resistant vehicle. Similarly campus officials at Hinds Community College in Mississippi, an institution enrolling approximately 11,000 students, acquired a repurposed grenade launcher through the program (Bauman, 2014).

Some campuses have supported the program. For example, Ohio State spokesman Dan Hedman emphasized the importance of being able to "respond at a moment's notice to any disaster—natural or man-made" (Kingkade & Svokos, 2014). Likewise, Florida International police chief Alexander Casas has argued that even though a department possesses military-grade equipment, officers know the difference between the role of campus police and the role of the military (Grasgreen, 2014).

However, the 1033 program has not been without criticism. For example, Georgia congressman Hank Johnson recently introduced the bipartisan Stop Militarizing Law Enforcement Act of 2014 to stem the flow of weapons from the military to police departments. As Johnson has stated, many departments are "quickly beginning to resemble paramilitary forces" (cited in Chasmar, 2014, para. 3). Specifically, a spokesperson for the congressman noted that "Ohio State

University recently acquired an MRAP [mine-resistant ambush protected vehicle]" and quipped that "apparently, college kids are getting too rowdy" (cited in Grasgreen, 2014, para. 9).

New state laws governing firearms on college and university campuses and litigation outcomes remain varied. Some have been seen as victories for gun control advocates, whereas others have not. Further, most state statutes governing firearms on college campuses apply only to public institutions, leaving private colleges to pass whatever regulation they choose. With no federal law providing guidance on the matter, states will continue to differ. If such federal legislation or regulations were forthcoming, would some states, such as Alaska, attempt to nullify the law? In response, would the federal government simply withhold Title IV funding from individual institutions?

Questions also remain regarding the arms held by local and campus police departments (Bauman, 2014). Many departments have participated in programs such as the Pentagon's 1033 program to acquire military arms and equipment, with many campus leaders arguing that such equipment is necessary for maintaining safe campus communities. However, incidents such as the 2011 pepper spraying of student protestors at the University of California, Davis, and the strong police response to the 2014 protests in Ferguson, Missouri, have drawn wide criticism and calls for rolling back police militarization. Indeed, some institutions are returning or considering returning equipment acquired under the program (Peagler, 2014; Ryman, 2014). It is unclear in which direction the pendulum will swing, let alone how far, as the debate appears to only be ratcheting up.

Conclusion

The U.S. Supreme Court's rulings in *District of Columbia v. Heller* and *McDonald v. City of Chicago* solidified an individual's right to bear arms under the Second Amendment, but the extent and application of the matter are left to the states to determine. Gun control legislation across the United States remains varied and divided, according to the political and social proclivities of a particular state. Although some states explicitly provide for concealed carry on college and university campuses, other states permit institutions of higher learning to make individual and varied determinations as to how concealed carry will function on their campuses. Litigation concerning such legislation, which is in its nascent stage, has largely favored overturning institutional bans on weapons. In New York, however, the state imposition on firearms has survived its first federal legal test, but appeal is likely and more remains to be seen.

Colleges and universities, large and small, public and private, are at the forefront of the discussion concerning firearms on campus, and rightfully so. Unspeakable tragedies have gripped higher education as institutions and their communities have faced the unnecessary and horrific deaths of students and staff as a result of campus violence. Higher education stands at a point of transition as a result and has certainly earned the right to participate as a salient voice in the public policy debate to help shape the contours of gun control legislation in the United States.

Acknowledgments

Portions of this chapter previously appeared in Hephner LaBanc, B., Melear, K. B., & Hemphill, B. (2014). The debate over campus gun control legislation. *Journal of College and University Law*, 40(3), 397–424. The authors appreciate the permission of the *Journal of College and University Law* to reprint content here.

Notes

1. California, Florida, Georgia, Illinois, Louisiana, Massachusetts, Michigan, Missouri, Nebraska, Nevada, New Jersey, New Mexico, New York, North Carolina, North Dakota, Ohio, Oklahoma, South Carolina, Tennessee, Texas, and Wyoming.

2. Alabama, Alaska, Arizona, Arkansas, Connecticut, Delaware, Hawaii, Indiana, Iowa, Kentucky, Maine, Maryland, Minnesota, Montana, New Hampshire, Pennsylvania, Rhode Island, South Dakota, Vermont, Virginia, Washington, and West Virginia.

3. Colorado, Idaho, Kansas, Mississippi, Oregon, Utah, and Wisconsin.

References

Act to Amend Part 3 of Article 4 of Chapter 11 of Title 16 of the Official Code of Georgia Annotated, (2013-2014).

Arkansas Act No. 226 (2013).

Bauman, D. (2014, September 11). On campus, grenade launchers, M-16s, and armored vehicles. *The Chronicle of Higher Education*. Retrieved from http://chronicle.com/article/On-Campus-Grenade-Launchers/148749/

Boise State University. (n.d.). *Boise State weapons on campus frequently asked questions*. Retrieved from http://security.boisestate.edu/wp-content/blogs.dir/1/files/2014/06/FAQ-Guns-on-Campus-as-of-June-26.pdf

Campbell, S. F. (2014, July 7). Will guns be allowed on campuses? *The Times-Herald*. Retrieved from http://www.times-herald.com/local/20140531-school-gun-carry-conflict

Chasmar, J. (2014, August 14). Democrat plans police anti-militarization bill amid Ferguson violence. *Washington Times*. Retrieved from http://www.washington-times.com/news/2014/aug/14/democrat-introduce-police-anti-militarization-bill/

DeSantis, N. (2014, March 7). Idaho lawmakers approve bill allowing guns on campuses. *The Chronicle of Higher Education*. Retrieved from http://www.chronicle.com/blogs/ticker/idaho-lawmakers-approve-bill-allowing-guns-on-campuses/73987

District of Columbia v. Heller, 554 U.S. 570 (2008).

Doubleday, J. (2013, September 11). Students oppose concealed-carry gun policy on campuses, survey finds. *The Chronicle of Higher Education*. Retrieved from http://chronicle.com/article/Students-Oppose/141543/

Drabold, W. (2014, July 8). Concealed-carry group sues Ohio State, says gun ban is too broad. *Columbus Dispatch*. Retrieved from http://www.dispatch.com/content/stories/local/2014/07/07/Concealed_carry_group_sues_Ohio_State_over_gun_ban.html

Federal Regulation, Chapter 52, SLA 13 (2013).

Flegenheimer, M. (2013, December 27). Final report on Sandy Hook killings sheds new light on gunman's isolation. *New York Times*. Retrieved from http://www.nytimes.com/2013/12/28/nyregion/with-release-of-final-sandy-hook-shooting-report-investigation-is-said-to-be-over.html?pagewanted=all

Florida Carry Inc. v. University of North Florida, 133 So. 3d (2013).

Frosch, D. (2012, September 22). University is uneasy as court ruling allows guns on campus. *New York Times*. Retrieved from http://www.nytimes.com/2012/09/23/education/guns-on-campus-at-university-of-colorado-causes-unease.html

Ga. HB 826(c)(6) (2013–2014).

Ga. Stat. Ann. § 16-11-127.1 (2014).

Graf, S. (2014, March 21). *Boise State sets policy as it prepares for guns on campus*. Retrieved from http://boisestatepublicradio.org/post/boise-state-sets-policy-it-prepares-guns-campus

Grasgreen, A. (2011, October 3). Guns come to campus. *Inside Higher Ed*. Retrieved from https://www.insidehighered.com/news/2011/10/03/concealed_carry_in_oregon_wisconsin_and_mississippi_means_changes_for_college_and_university_campuses

Grasgreen, A. (2012, March 6). Campus gun ban struck down. *Inside Higher Ed*. Retrieved from https://www.insidehighered.com/news/2012/03/06/state-supreme-court-rules-colorado-regents-cant-ban-guns

Grasgreen, A. (2014, August 25). College cops score defense supplies. *Politico*. Retrieved from http://www.politico.com/story/2014/08/defense-surplus-university-police-110323.html

Graves, B. (2011a, September 29). Oregon Court of Appeals rejects university system's ban on guns on campus. *Oregonian*. Retrieved from http://www.oregonlive.com/education/index.ssf/2011/09/oregon_court_of_appeals_reject.html

Graves, B. (2011b, November 8). Oregon University System will not appeal court decision allowing guns on campus. *Oregonian*. Retrieved from http://www.oregonlive.com/education/index.ssf/2011/11/oregon_university_system_will_1.html

Graves, B. (2012, March 2). Oregon State Board of Higher Education resorts to policy to ban guns on campus. *Oregonian*. Retrieved from http://www.oregonlive.com/education/index.ssf/2012/03/oregon_state_board_of_higher_e_7.html

Hatt, K. (2011). *Gun-shy originalism: The Second Amendment's original purpose in District of Columbia vs. Heller*. Retrieved from http://suffolklawreview.org/wp-content/uploads/2013/01/Hatt_Note_Macro.pdf

Hayes, S. (2014, January 6). USF policy change allows guns in cars on campus. *Tampa Bay Times*. Retrieved from http://www.tampabay.com/news/education/college/usf-policy-change-allows-guns-in-cars-on-campus/2159840

Idaho Senate Bill 1254 §4, 18-33-9(2) (2013–2014).

Kan. Stat. Ann. § 75-7c10 (2012).

Keller, J. (2011, September 28). Oregon Court of Appeals strikes down university system's ban on firearms. *The Chronicle of Higher Education*. Retrieved from http://chronicle.com/article/Oregon-Court-Strikes-Down/129184/

Kingkade, T. (2013, June 24). Arkansas colleges reject concealed carry on campus under loosened gun law. *Huffington Post*. Retrieved from http://www.huffingtonpost.com/2013/06/24/arkansas-concealed-carry-on-campus-colleges_n_3492425.html

Kingkade, T., Svokos, A. (2014, September 16). Campus police are stocking up on military-grade weapons. *Huffington Post*. Retrieved from http://www.huffingtonpost.com/2014/09/15/campus-police-weapons_n_5823310.html

Koplovitz, K. (2013, January 17). At last, real bipartisan leadership on gun control— Governor Cuomo takes the lead. *Huffington Post*. Retrieved from http://www.huffingtonpost.com/kay-koplovitz/new-york-gun-control_b_2495313.html

LaPoint, L. A. (2010). The up and down battle for concealed carry at public universities. *Journal of Student Affairs, 19*, 16–23.

Law Center to Prevent Gun Violence. (2014, January 7). *Victory in the courts: New York's new gun law largely upheld by federal district judge*. Retrieved from http://smartgunlaws.org/victory-in-the-courts-new-yorks-new-gun-law-upheld-by-federal-district-judge/

Laws taking effect Friday in Arkansas. (2013, August 16). Retrieved from http://www.arkansasmatters.com/story/d/story/laws-taking-effect-friday-in-arkansas/37417/qFDZ395-j021U36nx0E7yA

McDonald v. City of Chicago, 130 S. Ct. 3020 (2010).

Miss. Code Ann. § 97-37-1 (2011).

National Conference of State Legislatures. (2014). *Guns on campus: Overview*. Retrieved from http://www.ncsl.org/research/education/guns-on-campus-overview.aspx

New York Secure Ammunition and Firearms Enforcement (SAFE), Act S2230 (2013).

New York State Rifle and Pistol Association v. Cuomo, WL 6909955 (W.D.N.Y.) (2013).

Oregon Firearms v. Board of Higher Education, P264.3d 160, 165 (Or. 264 App. 2011).

Parker, B. (2013, December 18). Nullification-lite: Why states are stepping in to protect the Second Amendment from the feds. *Daily Caller*. Retrieved from http://dailycaller.com/2013/12/18/nullification-lite-why-states-are-stepping-in-to-protect-the-second-amendment-from-the-feds/

Peagler, A. (2014, September 17). HCC gets a grenade launcher through a military surplus program. *MSNewsNow*. Retrieved from http://www.msnewsnow.com/story/26562285/hcc-gets-a-gernade-launcher-through-the-10-33-program

Price, J. H., Thompson, A., Khubchandani, J., Dake, J., Payton, E., & Teeple, ...
(2014). University presidents' perceptions and practice regarding the carrying of
concealed handguns on college campuses. *Journal of American College Health,*
62(7), 461–469. doi:10.1080/07448481.2014.920336

Regents of the University of Colorado v. Students for Concealed Carry on Campus,
271 P.3d 496 (Colo. 2012).

Rezvani, A., Pupovac, J., Eads, D., & Fisher, T. (2014, September 2). *MRAPs and
bayonets: What we know about the Pentagon's 1033 Program.* Retrieved from
http://www.npr.org/2014/09/02/342494225/mraps-and-bayonets-what-we-know-
about-the-pentagons-1033-program

Richinick, M. (2014, July 1). *Georgia guns everywhere bill takes effect.* Retrieved
from http://www.msnbc.com/msnbc/georgia-guns-everywhere-bill-takes-effect

Russell, B. Z. (2014, February 3). Idaho college leaders oppose guns-on-campus bill, but
lawmakers press on anyway. *Spokesman-Review.* Retrieved from http://www.spokesman
.com/stories/2014/feb/03/idaho-college-leaders-oppose-guns-campus-bill-lawm/

Ryman, A. (2014, September 30). *ASU police plan to return surplus M-16 assault rifles.*
Retrieved from http://www.azcentral.com/story/news/local/tempe/2014/09/29/
asu-police-plan-return-surplus-m-16-assault-rifles/16448959/

Senate Bill 1254 §4, 18-33-9(2) (2013–2014).

Simms, C. (2014, May 29). *Update: Guns on campus? Georgia attorney general says
"no."* Retrieved from http://www.gpb.org/news/2014/05/29/update-guns-on-cam-
pus-georgia-attorney-general-says-%E2%80%9Cno%E2%80%9D

Skorton, D., & Altschuler, G. (2013, February 21). Do we really need more guns on
campus? *Forbes Magazine.* Retrieved from http://www.forbes.com/sites/college-
prose/2013/02/21/guns-on-campus/

State ex rel. Black v. State Board of Education, 33 Idaho 415, 196 P. 201 (1921).

Students for Concealed Carry on Campus. (n.d.). *About.* Retrieved from http://www
.concealedcampus.org/about

Tex. Bus. & Com. Code § 411.2032 (2013).

United States v. Miller, 307 U.S. 174 (1939).

University of Alaska. (2014). *Regents' policies.* Retrieved from https://www.alaska
.edu/bor/policy/02-09.pdf

U.S. Constitution, Second Amendment. (1791).

Utah Code, § 53-5a-102 (2013).

Williamson, J. (n.d.). *Memorandum: Possession of weapons on campus.* Retrieved
from http://www.police.uga.edu/documents/uga_weapons_policy.pdf

Wis. Stat. § 991.11.82.2a (2011).

Zuckerman, L. (2014, July 1). *Idaho college arms officers as law allowing guns on
campus takes effect.* Retrieved from http://www.huffingtonpost.com/2014/07/01/
idaho-college-weapons_n_5547107.html

ating an Emotionally
ealthy Community to Promote
Campus Safety

Maggie Balistreri-Clarke and Peter Meagher

College Students and Mental Health

During the last 20 years college and university counseling centers have seen large increases in both service utilization and severity of the mental illness symptoms presented (Kitzrow, 2003). These same college counseling centers have also moved from dealing primarily with developmental issues to "more severe psychological problems" (Kitzrow, 2003, p. 168). Gallagher (2006) reported that since 2004 college counseling center directors saw a rise in "self injury reports . . . demands for crisis counseling, . . . eating disorders, . . . sexual assault cases, . . . [and] reporting earlier childhood sexual abuse" (p. 5). The American College Health Association (2007) found in its spring 2006 college health survey ($N = 94,806$) that 38.5% of college students who took the survey reported feeling hopeless during the last school year, 27.5% reported feeling so sad it was difficult to function, and 7.3% had seriously considered attempting suicide.

It is difficult to pinpoint with certainty what has caused this increase. Kitzrow (2003) argued that it may be due to "cultural factors . . . [such as] divorce, family dysfunction . . . [or] early experimentation with drugs, alcohol and sex" (p. 171). Kitzrow also suggested that many serious mental illnesses, such as depression, bipolar disorder, or schizophrenia, commonly surface during the college years. Although accurate, neither of these explanations feels satisfactory. A final factor that Kitzrow acknowledged was that

> more students seeking [and being treated for mental health issues before coming to college] may also reflect a positive shift in atti-

tudes about mental health treatment and indicate a greater acceptance of treatment for mental health problems by the current
generation. (p. 171)

Gregg Heinselman, associate vice chancellor for student affairs
at the University of Wisconsin–River Falls (as reported by Guess,
2008), suggested two other factors: improved identification and
referral of students to counseling, and the phenomenon of "spiraling" (Guess, 2008, para. 14). Spiraling involves students coming to
campus "who were on medication in high school [and] who try to
get on with their lives without it once they reach the new college
environment" (p. 14). This is an intriguing theory and deserves further exploration. In sum, it is clear that students are entering college
presenting more serious symptoms of some forms of mental illness.

Mental Health and Violence—A Small Risk

For some, recent events have encouraged the belief that violence
on college campuses is on the rise. Indeed, pundits and scholars
are scrambling for an explanation for such tragic occurrences and
often place blame on individuals with mental health issues. These
attitudes raise a key question about the actual link between mental illness and violence. The connection is simultaneously complex
and subtle. Many scholars argue that mental health alone is a minor
factor, and that gender, socioeconomic status, and location play far
greater roles in everyday violence (Englander, 2007; Fazel & Grann,
2006; Rosenberg, 2014; Steadman et al., 1998). In addition, Steadman et al. (1998) found no difference in violence between those
with mental illness and those without. However, when substance
abuse is factored in as a co-occurring issue, the frequency of violence increases for both those with mental illness and those without,
and is actually twice the rate for those without a substance abuse
disorder (Steadman et al., 1998). As these authors noted, occurrence
of violence was lowest in their sample for those with schizophrenia,
followed by bipolar disorder and major depression. To summarize,
there is a "modest association" between mental illness and violence,
and this association is exacerbated significantly by substance abuse
(Stuart, 2003, p. 122).

Myths, Fears, and Stigma

Long before the high-profile cases at Virginia Tech and Northern
Illinois University, misperceptions and myths about mental illness
and how best to respond have existed. These misperceptions create
an environment that stigmatizes young people with mental illness
(Garske & Stewart, 1999). In one study of adolescents who had committed suicide, friends and family of the victims listed common barriers to seeking help (Moskos, Olson, Halbem, & Gray, 2007). These
included

> ➢ believing nothing could help;
> ➢ having the perception that seeking help was a sign of weakness
>   or failure;
> ➢ being reluctant to admit having problems;
> ➢ denying they have problems; and
> ➢ being too embarrassed to seek help.

Clearly, these beliefs prevent young people from seeking the mental
health assistance that could potentially save their lives.

Adverse Childhood Experiences and Our Students

Students arrive at college with experiences that have shaped them
in many ways—from subtle to profound. Campus professionals with
information on the precursors to maladaptive behaviors and mental
health issues can be more empathetic and can better respond to these
students. One groundbreaking body of literature seeks to understand
the impact of adverse childhood experiences (ACEs) on long-term
health outcomes, including depression, alcohol and drug use, suicide
attempts, smoking, and risk for intimate partner violence (Felitti et
al., 1998). In a study that included over 9,508 individuals, more than
half experienced at least one ACE and nearly one in five experienced
three or more ACEs. The researchers found that a direct relationship
between the number of ACEs an individual experiences and his or
her risk for developing one of the negative outcomes.

Prior to the ACEs study, risk factors had been studied individually in relation to their impact on various life outcomes. The ACEs

study was designed to look at the interaction of risk factors with outcomes. The ACEs study reviewed data collected from a survey of 9,508 health plan members and correlated member responses to health information obtained through clinical interviews (Dong et al., 2004). The ACEs can be grouped into the following categories: abuse (psychological, sexual, physical), neglect (emotional and physical), witnessing domestic violence, parental marital discord, and living with substance-abusing, mentally ill, or criminal household members (Dong et al., 2004). Individuals were then assessed using childhood exposures to the ACEs and physical factors associated with the leading causes of death. These included smoking, severe obesity, physical inactivity, depressed mood, suicide attempts, alcoholism, and drug abuse.

The results are stunning and have far-ranging implications for the student development professional. The findings offer a number of simple takeaway messages. First, ACEs are very common. As noted earlier, over half of the respondents (52%) reported having at least one ACE (Felitti et al., 1998). The most common ACE was exposure to substance abuse, and the least common was exposure to criminal activity (3.4%). Second, the factors were highly interrelated. For example, growing up with parents with alcoholism was related to other experiences, such as exposure to emotional, physical, or sexual abuse. As the number of individuals in the home who abused alcohol increased, so too did the amount of abuse. Consequently, the research team developed an "ACE score," which is related to one's risk of experiencing various physical and emotional issues. The higher the ACE score, the more likely other risks are to arise.

ACEs, Mental Health, and Intimate Partner Violence

The presence of ACEs is highly relevant for the college-age population because this is the time when the impact of a traumatic environment in childhood, in terms of mental health and violence, may surface. Indeed, many common mental health and violence-related issues are highly connected to the amount of childhood exposure to trauma and common stressors facing college students. For example, people who are exposed to four or more ACE categories have a substantial increase (4- to 12-fold) in risk for substance abuse, depression, and suicide attempts (Felitti et al., 1998). Although experiencing any of the ACEs increases the risk of negative outcome, these negative health outcomes are not inevitable.

Exposure to abuse in the home in particular affects the risk of becoming a victim or perpetrator of intimate partner violence. *Abuse* was defined as an individual experiencing physical or sexual abuse, or witnessing the physical abuse of a family member. Experiencing any one of these forms of abuse made it twice as likely that women would become a victim of violence and that men would perpetrate violence. For those who had experienced all three of the factors, the likelihood of women becoming victims of violence increased by 3.5%. The likelihood that men would perpetuate violence increased by 3.8% (Whitfield, Anda, Dube, & Felitti, 2003).

For those who work on college campuses, the specter of interpersonal violence has been a vexing challenge. Interpersonal violence often goes unreported, and its prevalence is common and devastating. We know that women and men both experience and perpetuate interpersonal violence. However, in regard to a whole host of factors, women experience more intimate partner violence and related issues. Black et al. (2011), in the National Intimate and Sexual Violence Survey (NISVS), reported 3 in 10 women and 1 in 10 men experienced sexual assault, physical assault, and/or stalking. In addition, these authors reported that women were more likely than men to experience serious harm and were more likely to experience a consequence of the violence, including fear, concern for their safety, post-traumatic stress disorder (PTSD) symptoms, or injury. Lastly, both men and women reported needing crisis line, advocacy, housing, or legal services, and women were more likely to miss a day of school or work.

Of those who experience intimate partner violence, women between the ages of 20 and 24 are at greatest risk (Rennison & Welchans, 2000). In this age group, homicide is the fourth leading cause of death among women (Centers for Disease Control and Prevention, 2010), and, for more than one third of all women who are murdered (39.3%), the perpetrator is an intimate partner (Catalano, 2013).

The research just presented outlines the challenges students bring to campus, the rise of mental illness in college students, and the relationship between violence and mental illness. As noted, there is only a modest association between violence and mental illness. The remainder of this chapter explores a proactive approach to identifying students who are displaying mental health symptoms and to connecting them to professional help. The key to this strategy is to create emotionally healthy campus climates. The case will be made for this as both an efficient and effective approach. As Sara Abelson of Active Minds (AM) (www.activeminds.org) explains, "There is a common set of strategies to build a healthy campus community, and these efforts should have positive impacts across all different threats" (personal communication, June 4, 2014).

Creating an Emotionally Healthy Campus

After the mass school shooting at an elementary school in Connecticut in December 2012, an interdisciplinary group of school violence prevention researchers and practitioners and associated organizations issued a position statement. The joint statement included a call to promote wellness and address mental health needs of all community members, while also responding to community safety (Curry School of Education, 2012). Promoting wellness as a key factor in promoting campus safety focuses attention on creating an emotionally healthy campus climate that fosters the well-being of all members of the campus community. This involves creating communities of care that send messages of value, respect, mattering, and connectedness to all and call for the creation of systems and behaviors that bring these ideals to reality.

There are multiple benefits to be gained from targeting efforts toward building a healthy campus community. A healthy campus community is one in which high priority is placed on creating conditions where all may thrive. As Reich (n.d.) explained, this focus on student well-being is not about promoting a superficial experience of being happy or even feeling happy, but rather about those insights that are more to the heart and purpose of higher education. Well-being, or what Keyes (2002) called "flourishing," involves a "sustainable quality of purpose that underlies our sense of self, our motivation to persist, our trust in agency and our responsibility to act for the common good" (p. 14).

Student well-being is linked to qualities that are foundational for learning and human capacity building (Finley, n.d.). The researchers with the Healthy Minds Study, directed by Daniel Eisenberg at the University of Michigan, also link student health and well-being to increased student success and retention ("Gatekeeper," 2013). Increased student retention benefits both the individual and the institution. Beyond the economic benefits are those that emerge from fulfilling higher education's purpose of promoting student learning and success. For those whose more immediate concern is campus safety, the benefits increase exponentially when the individual student's well-being promotes an increased sense of responsibility to act for the common good.

Efforts to create an emotionally healthy campus climate are grounded in many assumptions, beliefs, and strategies that are shared by those focused on promoting campus safety, preventing sexual assault, preventing suicide, and preventing alcohol and drug abuse. A comprehensive approach can build strong campus partnerships and generate synergy among strategies for targeting different issues—all of which can lead to assisting students before they reach the point of crisis.

A Strategic Planning Approach

To bring about effective and meaningful change, a campuswide, strategic planning approach offers an excellent framework for creating an emotionally healthy campus climate. There are many advantages to this approach. First, a strategic planning approach will directly tie healthy-campus efforts to higher education's primary mission of promoting student learning and success and ensuring persistence to graduation. Second, this approach will seek to engage all members of the campus community, thereby promoting a deeper level of commitment and ownership. Finally, a strategic planning approach will involve creating measures that can be used to generate specific strategies, action plans, and means for gauging the progress of a campus toward the specific wellness goals. Specific components to be addressed in a strategic planning approach include the following practices:

1. *Create a sense of urgency.* Every campus has competing priorities. Therefore it is important to build a sense of urgency (Kotter, 2008), buy-in, and importance around the goal of creating an emotionally healthy campus climate. In an effort to develop a sense of urgency around students' emotional

needs, Erik Albinson, vice president for student affairs at Coe College, gave a presentation to Coe's board of trustees on the mental health of today's college students. According to Albinson, this led to a greater awareness of the emotional needs of today's college students on the part of both board of trustee members and the other vice presidents attending the meeting (Albinson, personal communication, June 23, 2015). This, in turn, raised the level of support and expanded buy-in for a sharper focus on student well-being as a theme in the college's strategic planning.

2. *Create a guiding coalition.* In his book *Leading Change*, Kotter (2008) made a strong case for creating a guiding coalition made up of diverse members. On college campuses, such a coalition or chartered team, would involve a diverse group of students, faculty, and staff. The purpose of creating such a group is to build ownership for needed change, to develop a deeper understanding of issues, and to generate more creative and effective action plans.

   Although a guiding coalition would ideally mean a cross-college group reflecting an institution's deep commitment to promoting campus mental health, this approach can be used at any level within higher education. A residence hall director could gather a diverse group interested in strengthening the emotional health of residents within a specific residence hall. Such a group could include resident assistants, hall residents, and a supportive faculty or staff member outside of the residence life department.

   Students involved in campus organizations dedicated to promoting campus mental health, such as AM, could invite interested faculty and staff members to join them and thereby expand their base of support and heighten visibility for their efforts.

   With the proliferation of behavioral intervention teams, many campuses already have a structure for teams intended to guide violence prevention campus efforts. The JED Foundation, whose mission is "to promote emotional health and prevent suicide among college and university students" (www.thejedfoundation.org), offers a free downloadable booklet entitled *Balancing Safety and Support on Campus: A Guide for Campus Teams*. The intent of this resource is to provide practical and accessible guidance for the creation and management of teams who serve as guiding coalitions around violence prevention efforts.

3. *Create an action plan with measurable goals.* Too often higher education professionals will launch a strategy that appears to hold promise before agreeing on desired outcomes. It is important to first agree on what success will look like and how the college community will know it is making progress. Creating measurable goals will serve to focus strategies on specific desired outcomes. Taking time to agree on specific measurable goals will engage team members in important discussions about which strategies will have the biggest impact, while building a sense of buy-in from all constituents. This process of working collaboratively to set measurable goals will engender a deeper understanding of the most critical issues and a greater commitment to strategies tied to specific, agreed-upon outcomes.

The American College Health Association's "Healthy Campus 2020" index (n.d.) includes potential health measures that can be used as a tool for developing and monitoring health goals and objectives. These measures include student retention, graduation and turnover rates, student satisfaction, and availability of suicide prevention services.

Edgewood College in Madison, Wisconsin, makes use of both homegrown and nationally normed survey instruments to capture data on measures such as connectedness and belonging. Survey items include, "I feel a sense of belonging on campus," and "There is at least one faculty or staff member to whom I can go for assistance." The survey responses can be separated out by year, resident status, gender, race, and so on to help the campus focus energy and attention on strengthening a sense of connectedness and belonging for different populations on campus. Edgewood has created a dashboard to track measures such as satisfaction and engagement, which can be indicators of student well-being on campus.

The following concepts can serve as a framework for creating emotionally healthy campus communities and can serve as components of the strategic plan.

Shape the Campus Environment

The brother-in-law of one of this chapter's authors recently described the experience of taking his son for college admissions visits. On each campus, within a relatively short time, the son would begin commenting about whether he could "see himself" at that campus. As the father described it, "It was as if there were something in the air" (P. Clarke, personal communication, January 25, 2014). That "something in the air" is what Strange and Banning (2001) defined as the *campus environment*.

Campus environments are created by passive means, such as the upkeep of buildings, campus banners, and the availability of spaces students find attractive. Campus environments or campus cultures can also be shaped by active means, such as by promoting messages through various media, by emphasizing values, and by implementing policies and practices that encourage or punish behaviors.

Among strong communities, Strange and Banning (2001) described a synergy of components, where members can pursue a common purpose over time in ways that are sustained by the shared characteristics and collective qualities of community members. Certain forms of environmental dimensions seem to support the development of community more than others. An environment specifically designed to promote an emotionally healthy campus culture will include multiple messages about the need to care for one's self. In addition, there will be a high expectation that members of this community are responsible for the well-being of others. Such an environment will have low barriers to connecting with personal counseling and health services and will normalize help-seeking behaviors through messages delivered by student leaders and social media.

Nurture Connectedness

Promoting a feeling of connectedness is foundational to creating emotionally healthy communities. According to Whitlock, Wyman, and Barreira (2012) connectedness is best understood as a psychological state of being that reflects a sense of closeness, embeddedness, and visibility to individuals and groups. Additionally, it is a relationship system through which perceptions are generated and norms are translated. For this chapter, it is particularly crucial to note that connectedness is linked to decreased rates of mental illness and can serve as a protective factor against suicide (Whitlock et al., 2012). Such decreases are potentially due to various relational outcomes that are introduced by instilling connectedness as a value.

Campus environments that strive to create a feeling of connectedness among all students will move beyond a traditional sense of school spirit, often more closely tied to the prowess of athletic teams than to the well-being of students. Connectedness involves generating experiences of affirmation, respect, and caring about and for all members of the campus community. Higher connectedness across social spheres may confer benefits by exposing young people to normative social influences that encourage positive coping practices, such as seeking formal and informal support and reducing maladaptive coping practices (e.g., drinking).

Whitlock et al. (2012) explained that connectedness can arise from not only *interpersonal* experiences but also *intrapersonal* ones. Interpersonal connectedness is found most obviously on any given campus in countless relationships, where faculty members reach out to students to express concern or encouragement, where resident assistants seek out a student who appears to be struggling, or where a student leader takes time to mentor a new student.

Beyond individual interactions, Whitlock et al. (2012) explained that individuals form deep attachments to their internal understanding of themselves through narratives and beliefs about their lives and also through abstract concepts, such as justice or compassion. These intrapersonal narratives and core beliefs can play a powerful role in shaping emotions, behaviors, and attitudes. They can also mediate receptivity to connectedness to others by acting as a filter for external events. Connectedness to others or to core ideas may serve as a protective factor to help students more positively appraise their relationships and buffer them from feelings of aloneness that can lead to psychological distress.

A campus community that seeks to promote both interpersonal and intrapersonal connectedness will support and reward outreach to and caring for individuals. The creation of an ethos of care will generate a culture that supports policies, practices, and structures that nurture connectedness for all students. For example, faculty will be recognized for creating safe and inclusive classrooms, and student leaders who serve as positive bridges for other students will be held up as exemplars. Staff members who reach out to students who have been prone to early departure from campus will be supported and recognized for their efforts.

Connectedness can be promoted through the intentional promotion and study of values and ideals, such as partnership and compassion. Every institution employs language to reflect the mission, vision, and/or highest ideals of that school. Efforts to bring about meaningful change will be more effective if grounded in the mission, culture, and language of the institution.

For example, Edgewood College maintains five values grounded in the Dominican heritage that is central to the college's culture: truth, justice, compassion, partnership, and community. Each year the college centers on a different value as a way to build connectedness among all members of the college community. Acceptance letters welcome students as members of a class representing the Dominican value that will be the focus for the coming year, such as the "Class of Compassion." New student orientation sessions named for the year's value engage students in small-group exercises led by student leaders, faculty, and staff members. By engaging students early in exercises centered on what the values mean and how one would act if guided by this value, a sense of connectedness is cultivated. This sends an early message that strong relationships and an expectation of connectedness are at the heart of the campus culture. This type of early engagement sets the expectation for connectedness and a sense of responsibility to and for each other as an essential part of being an Edgewood College student. As noted previously, promoting a sense of connectedness has many potential benefits, such as buffering students from feelings of isolation that can lead to psychological distress.

Focus on Thriving

With the rise of behavioral intervention teams, more community members are trained to be alert for students who may be at risk of harming themselves or others. A positive outcome of these efforts is heightened awareness within the larger college community of the need to pay attention to students who may be displaying symptoms of potentially violent behaviors. A critical component of violence prevention is a campus community whose members pay attention to and share information about students who may be showing signs of distress. However, the main purpose of most behavioral intervention teams is to gather information on and generate an appropriate response to those who may be displaying behaviors that could lead to harm to self or others. Therefore, behavioral intervention teams may be limited due to their essentially and necessarily reactive approach to campus safety.

Keyes (2002) offered a more positive and promising framework that moves away from a "mental illness versus mental health" continuum to a more robust perspective. This concept is illustrated in Figure 3.1, where the horizontal axis represents mental health symptoms ranging from severe to none. The vertical axis represents mental health ranging from languishing to flourishing.

Students in the top-left quadrant have mental illness symptoms, yet they are flourishing, whereas students in the bottom-right quadrant are languishing but have no symptoms of illness (Keyes, 2002).

Applying this approach to the creation of an emotionally healthy campus climate would focus on moving as many students as possible to the upper-right quadrant. This process would begin by creating conditions in which all students could thrive with no mental illness symptoms. It would create a more robust understanding of student well-being. For example, campus discussions centered on what it means for students to flourish with no mental illness symptoms could bring about a shared understanding of what it means for all students to flourish. This framework could also be used as an educational tool to discuss what is meant by "mental illness symptoms" as separate from the larger category of mental illness.

A specific outcome measure for moving students to the upper-right quadrant could be decreasing the number of students who are hospitalized for mental health crises. Success for this outcome would require specific action steps to reach students *before* they reach a crisis point.

Figure 3.1   Corey Keyes Model (2002)

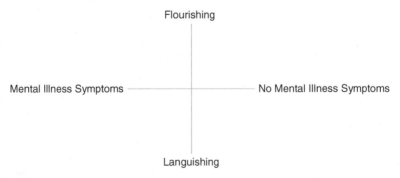

Create Sense of Shared Ownership for Student Well-being

Creating safer communities starts with a sense of collective responsibility for safeguarding the vulnerable and building collective resilience. This involves cultivating the shared belief that *everyone* within a campus community is responsible for the greater good. This notion of shared responsibility for the well-being of all is at the heart of what it means to be a community. Strange and Banning (2001) stated the following in their text on creating campus communities that work:

> [C]rucial to this quality of successful communities is the measure of "responsible concern" members demonstrate, including not looking away when a member is in need, a known set of community values and the obligation to confront a member when he deviates from these values. (p. 163)

This concept of shared responsibility for the well-being of all students serves to shift the focus away from the view of health professionals as the sole stoppers of threatening behavior (Whitlock et al., 2012) toward the belief that *everyone* within a community has a stake in maintaining the well-being of all members. Empowering students, faculty, and staff with the tools to identify a student in need, to know how to intervene, and to feel motivated and confident to take action is at the heart of educational and prevention efforts aimed at student well-being. The core beliefs, assumptions, and goals are the same—whether the focus is on preventing sexual misconduct, creating social justice allies, or reaching a student before a violent act seems like the only available solution.

An excellent example of how both in-person and virtual methods are used to spread this ethos of shared responsibility can be seen at Butler University, where Levester Johnson, vice president for student affairs, introduces new students to the three elements of Butler's "Community of Care" during new student orientation: (a) Take personal responsibility; (b) support others who are trying to do the same; and (c) have each other's back. This message is reinforced through Butler's Twitter hashtag, #CommunityofCare. On Butler's Twitter page students are connected to playful videos and tweets that reinforce Butler's Community of Care message of shared responsibility.

Faculty members at Edgewood College are encouraged to take three specific steps to reinforce a message of shared responsibility for the well-being of students: (a) Notice when students may be struggling; (b) reach out to express concern; and (c) connect students to resources. One of the authors delivers this message to faculty and staff in multiple settings, such as during new employee orientations and in intercollege assemblies. This simple formula is intended to offer a clear message and specific action steps toward creating an ethos of shared responsibility for the well-being of all students.

Strategies That Work

The most effective strategies for creating emotionally healthy campus communities will be embedded in a strategic approach, focus on the environment, nurture connectedness, focus on thriving, and create a sense of shared responsibility for the well-being of all students.

As mentioned earlier, a critical element of this effort will be a visible and vocal commitment to creating an emotionally healthy campus climate from the highest levels of campus leadership. Initiatives for promoting student wellness and emotional health can be generated at any level on campus, from a college-sanctioned coalition to a strategy created by a single student.

An excellent example of a strategic, robust, campuswide approach can be seen in the Healthy Campus Community Initiative at Simon Fraser University. The mission of this initiative is "to engage and enable staff, faculty, students, administrators and community partners to work collectively toward creating campus conditions that enhance well-being and success for all" (Simon Fraser University, n.d.). Gustavus Adolphus College's Wellbeing Initiative is another example of a comprehensive approach to emotional health. Gustavus offers Be-U group coaching opportunities to students, staff, and faculty to promote "optimal living . . . that support[s] personal discovery, holistic health, and lifelong learning" (M. Krause, personal communication, October 16, 2014).

An example of a student-led initiative that targets the environment comes from Grinnell College, where a student conceived and directed a project called the "Wellness Lounge." Houston Dougharty, vice president for student affairs, reported that this project has created great traction for campus mental health efforts (personal communication, July 2, 2014). According to Dougharty, the grant-funded Wellness

Lounge, located on the second floor of the Campus Center, was once a nondescript study nook and now has been transformed into a "funky and very comfy place for students to stop in, gather, and study." They have tea available, which students drink while they relax in the massage chair, work on a jigsaw puzzle, chat with a friend, or check their Facebook. Students designed it and maintain it. Dougharty sees this as a terrific addition to an intense and stressful campus and reports that many students use it daily. He added that even faculty and staff stop in, which serves to expand the reach of this student-generated project.

Coe College's vice president for student affairs, Erik Albinson, is shifting the emphasis from bystander training to weaving a student wellness and positive psychology foundation into the college's leadership development programs. This shift teaches student leaders positive coping strategies, promotes the early identification of issues, builds knowledge of how to respond, and creates the motivation to take action. Using positive psychology as the basis for developing student leaders is an excellent example of nurturing connectedness and deepening a sense of mutual responsibility for others on campus.

Strategies for Outreach and Intervention

In a review of the research on help-seeking for mental health on college campuses, Eisenberg, Hunt, and Speer (2012) observed that the most common intervention strategies fall into three categories: (a) Stigma reduction and educational outreach programs, (b) screening and linkage programs, and (c) gatekeeper training programs. These categories provide a helpful way to organize the types of strategies seen on many college campuses. In addition to the goal of connecting students who may be displaying mental illness symptoms to appropriate resources, many of these strategies target the environment, promote connectedness, and send clear messages of shared responsibility for the well-being of all students.

Stigma reduction and educational outreach programs

What stops college students with mental health concerns from seeking help in a timely manner? Eisenberg et al. (2012) explained that, as reflected in most theoretical models of help-seeking behavior, researchers consistently find that "negative attitudes and beliefs are significant barriers to help-seeking among college students" (p. 225). Therefore, many college campuses center their mental health educational outreach efforts on reducing the stigma that may prevent students from seeking treatment.

These stigma-reduction initiatives have the added benefit of also raising the general sense of well-being among all students. As discussed earlier in this chapter, creating conditions in which *all* students may thrive promotes student learning, fosters a deeper sense of connectedness, and promotes an ethos of care and responsibility for the common good. A common method for reaching out to the general student population is through educational outreach programs designed to diminish stigma reduction, raise awareness, and promote advocacy for various mental health issues.

Rather than passively serving the students who walk through their doors, many professional campus health and counseling services staff see educational outreach as a critical part of their mission. Typical programs will use a variety of methods to reach students, such as messaging campaigns, speakers, and public art displays. In addition to the work of healthcare professionals, students are often engaged in educational outreach efforts as an effective means to both expand the reach of programs and deepen the level of awareness of student leaders involved in program planning.

For example, AM is a nonprofit organization started in 2003 whose mission is to encourage an open dialogue among college students about mental health that will enhance education efforts and self-help initiatives. Through its support of more than 400 chapters on college campuses across the country, AM works to change the culture on campuses and in the community. The chapters sponsor events and programs primarily to raise awareness and provide advocacy training for mental health issues. AM provides chapters with educational content (i.e., latest statistics on mental health) to use on campus. This information can be tailored to the needs of each campus. Through the development of resources, such as brochures, fact sheets, or wallet cards, information on topics such as how to support a friend or how to recognize when a friend is struggling has become widely available.

Jessica Burman is a therapist with Counseling and Psychological Services at Cabrini College. She described Cabrini's AM chapter as one of the most active groups on campus—a group that enhances events already happening on campus. For example, Cabrini College is sponsoring a campuswide walk on the theme of homelessness. The AM students will place inspirational quotes along the walking path along with statistics that demonstrate the relationship between mental illness and homelessness (J. Burman, personal communication, October 14, 2014).

AM places special emphasis on developing student leaders. Madeline Coutu is the president of the AM chapter at Cabrini College. She is also a member of the National Student Advisory Committee. She explained:

> My experience with Active Minds has been life-changing and so important to my development professionally and my leadership development. Active Minds has, in many ways, solidified that my true passions lie in advocating for mental health reform and for those who suffer with various mental illnesses, as well as being educated about mental health issues. Active Minds also provided me with the place to feel fulfilled. I was and am doing something with myself. I am making a change and a difference. (M. Coutu, personal communication, October 19, 2014)

Coutu's enthusiasm for her experience as a leader committed to mental health advocacy is a reflection of AM's goal of nurturing the next generation of mental health advocates

Another source of support offered to campus chapters is the AM Speakers Bureau. Speakers willing to tell their stories serve as an effective outreach strategy. Research has clearly demonstrated that personal contact with someone with a lived experience of mental illness is an effective way to reduce stigma (Corrigan, Druss, & Perlick, 2014). Speaker events often lead to opportunities for audience members to share their own stories, which can serve to normalize mental illness and help-seeking within a campus culture.

In addition to bringing in outside speakers, creating opportunities for students to share their personal stories is an excellent stigma-reduction strategy. For example, "Night to Stop the Suffering" is a regular event at Cabrini College during which students can share personal stories about their struggles with mental illness. This event offers an opportunity for students to talk about their difficulties with stressful situations, such as dealing with an abusive relationship or coming out as gay. As part of their sponsorship of the event, the AM chapter always provides a "party bag" of favors, including things such as self-care items and contact information for connecting with professionals in Counseling and Psychological Services or local suicide hotlines and warmlines. Typically, students will offer spontaneous endorsement regarding the help they received through counseling services, even naming the counselors who helped them. According to Burman, who serves as the AM chapter adviser, these genuine testimonials affirm the message that students do not need to suffer alone and normalize help-seeking as a part of the college experience (J. Burman, personal communication, October 14, 2014).

Larger-scale public art events have the advantage of reaching many students in a short period of time and generating campuswide conversations about mental health topics. "Send Silence Packing" is a powerful example of the type of public awareness programming that AM sponsors. Over 1,100 college students commit suicide each year. As a dramatic illustration of this startling statistic, Send Silence Packing is a traveling exhibition that involves the placing of 1,100 backpacks in a high-traffic area on campus. More than 300 of the backpacks come with personal stories of college students lost to suicide. Sara Abelson, senior director of programs for AM, explains that "this program serves as a focal point for generating conversations about the role of everyone on campus in preventing suicide, connecting students to needed mental health resources, and building momentum for mental health promotion" (personal communication, September 8, 2014). Programs that build an ethos of community care and connectedness can reinforce the message of shared responsibility for the well-being of all students.

Screening and linkage programs

This category of outreach programs offers screening that identifies students in distress and then links them to appropriate services. Screening and linkage programs have evolved to take advantage of both face-to-face and virtual methods of reaching out to students. Screening and linkage programs may also serve as a way to scan the environment for students who may be languishing and/or displaying mental illness symptoms.

One program that offers both in-person and online screening is CollegeResponse, which is used by approximately 670 schools annually. The in-person version of CollegeResponse is held on the first Thursday of the first full week in October, in conjunction with National Depression Screening Day. At the campus events, students are invited to take a brief survey in which they self-screen for issues such as depression, bipolar disorder, and anxiety disorders. The surveys are reviewed by a healthcare professional looking for elevated risk of depression or other mental health concerns. Students who score positive for increased risk are given referral information for further evaluation and treatment if needed.

Megan Cobb, director of personal counseling services at Edgewood College, has been involved in National Depression Screening Day events on several campuses. She noted that many schools will host depression screening programs in large spaces, helping to raise awareness of signs and symptoms of depression and drawing attention to the opportunity to be screened. However, for this type of event it is important to balance openness with the need for privacy, and some larger locations may not foster a sense of confidentiality. Cobb has also been involved with schools whose screening programs are held right in the college's counseling center. Although this has the benefit of bringing students into the counseling center, this strategy could miss the opportunity for creating greater awareness and normalizing screening, which is an advantage of hosting the event in a more public space. She recommended conducting the event in a public space where private rooms are available for counselors and healthcare professionals to meet with students to discuss their survey results and conduct further assessment for students whose surveys indicate elevated risk.

At Cabrini College, students from AM partner with Counseling and Psychological Services to promote National Depression Screening Day. Students offer handouts with statistics and use social media to advertise the event. Burman sees the AM chapter as "a great mouthpiece and a great advocate for our services" (personal communication, October 14, 2014). Her observation is that students may go first to other students for support and the AM students will connect them to the mental health professionals on campus.

Given the amount of time that the typical college student spends online, outreach efforts that connect with students electronically have a number of advantages, such as 24/7 accessibility. Online screening tools may also be less threatening and offer students a deeper sense of privacy. An online version of the screening tool used at campus events is also available to students (www.HelpYourselfHelpOthers.org). This tool was developed by Mental Health Screening, the nonprofit organization that pioneered National Depression Screening Day in 1991.

An assessment of the National Depression Day online screening tool was conducted in 2009 by Robert Aseltine, director of the Institute for Public Health at the University of Connecticut Health Center. Aseltine found that of those who completed the depression screening tool, 55% of participants sought depression treatment within 3 months of screening (cited in Grohol, 2009, para. 8).

Gatekeeper training programs

Gatekeeper training (GKT) programs train campus members who are in a position to observe behavior, who have contact with resources and campus professionals, and who could be expected to provide initial outreach to someone who may be struggling. Lipson (2014) defined *gatekeeper training programs* as

> universal, primary prevention programs that aim to: (i) increase knowledge about mental health problems and the ability of gatekeepers to recognize and appropriately intervene in the face of such problems, and, as a result, (ii) increase the help-seeking behaviors of the target population. (p. 309)

GKT programs are conducted on many college campuses as a promising outreach strategy for suicide prevention and for more general mental health issues, such as anxiety and depression (Eisenberg et al., 2012). Some form of GKT can be seen in typical resident assistant training or in training programs designed to encourage faculty or staff to recognize warning signs, to reach out to students who may be showing signs of mental health issues, and to connect students to a higher level of assistance.

The rise in popularity of GKT programs may be due in part to the proliferation of behavioral intervention teams, which emphasize early identification of students who may be showing signs of harm to self or others. The surgeon general's 2012 *National Strategy for Suicide Prevention* (U.S. Department of Health and Human Services, 2012) identified GKT programs as a promising practice, thus raising the popularity and profile of these programs on campuses nationwide.

Although GKT programs are growing in popularity, their rapid implementation comes before the research on effectiveness has been fully developed regarding actually linking students to professional help. In a comprehensive review of GKT for adolescents and young adults, Lipson (2014) found that "the causal impact of GKT is sometimes exaggerated" (p. 318) and that there is little evidence these programs actually lead to getting students in distress to professional help. The program review also suggests the positive results of training may diminish over time.

Lipson, Speer, Brunwasser, Hahn, and Eisenberg (2014) conducted a follow-up study, this time of 32 colleges and universities conducting the GKT program, Mental Health First Aid (MHFA), which at the time was a 12-hour program. This study found that although there was not an increase in connecting students within the broader community to professional mental health assistance, there was evidence of positive effects on those who were trained. Following MHFA training, trainees were more likely to seek professional mental health assistance. There was also an increase in the self-perceived knowledge and self-efficacy of resident assistants. Although it is tempting to conclude that one approach could be to expand the GKT programs to a wider population to extend the benefits to more students, Lipson et al. (2014) also found that the effect of the MHFA training was stronger for those resident assistants who started with higher baseline knowledge. The study concludes that although there were personal benefits for the resident assistants who were trained, a new iteration of GKT models may be needed to improve effectiveness. As Lipson et al. (2014) noted, "Trainees may need a more sustained learning process with repeated opportunities to practice skills and discuss gatekeeping experiences" (p. 618). The study also concludes that peers other than resident assistants may be more effective gatekeepers; although a resident assistant's previous experience may be an advantage, the level of authority that comes with the role may be a barrier to actually linking students in distress to professional help.

As an alternative to GKT programs that require an extensive time commitment, Victor Schwartz, MD, medical director for The JED Foundation (www.jedfoundation.org), proposed a different approach. He posited that a different level of training—one that is appropriate to the level of action that needs to be taken—could be more effective. Dr. Schwartz contended that many lengthy GKT programs actually do too much. The more detailed and complicated the training, the less likely those trained are to intervene. Through simpler and more intuitive training, those trained are more likely to intervene. Dr. Schwartz drew a comparison with other types of intervention training. For example, with more extensive CPR training, those trained have an increased fear that they will do something wrong.

Dr. Schwartz noted that "you actually don't need a lot of sophistication, but rather what is helpful is having a basic idea of what needs to be done" (personal communication, October 13, 2014). He explained that for this type of training, you will lose people after half an hour. According to Dr. Schwartz, current GKT programs give too much information—they make it seem as if you need special knowledge, which is having the wrong impact.

The JED Foundation, whose mission is to promote emotional health and prevent suicide among college and university students, is developing a GKT program with this simpler approach. Dr. Schwartz explains that it is important for administrators to trust their instincts and intuitions. He offers a simple two-step process: (a) Offer a simple presentation and (b) give frequent reminders. For the reminders, his suggestion is that not a lot of content is needed. Initial training will have an impact for one or two weeks. He explains that if you want people to remember past that time, you need to offer small reminders—perhaps include items in school publications as a way to keep the information fresh.

Further Considerations

Reflecting on the sparse evidence for the effectiveness of many current interventions for college students in distress, Eisenberg et al. (2012) encouraged the use of research on other health behaviors for strategies that may be more effective in generating behavioral change. In the study by Lipson et al. (2014), the effectiveness of GKT programs centers on actual help-seeking as the desired outcome. However, perhaps this is too high of an initial standard. As in other areas of health education, merely being aware that one may have a problem may not result in actively doing anything about it as the very next step.

Motivational interviewing (MI) is an approach used to address health issues such as alcohol abuse and smoking. The MI framework offers a progression of stages of change that transition from precontemplation to contemplation, preparation, action, and maintenance of the decision. Using this framework, if a student who is experiencing mental illness symptoms was to be approached by a concerned person, such as a trained gatekeeper, helping the student become aware that others are concerned may move that student into precontemplation. This is the first stage of making the decision to take action to address the problem, such as seeking professional help (Prochaska & DiClemente, 1983). Although reaching students before they reach the point of crisis and connecting them to the appropriate level of assistance are the ultimate goals, it may be unrealistic to think that one or two initial interactions with a concerned resident assistant would be enough to move a student who is struggling with mental illness to seek professional assistance. However, despite this truth, this action still holds great value. A resident assistant approaching others with his or her concern may also work toward creating a sense of urgency in the students, another effective MI approach. By creating a deeper sense of urgency among students who would benefit from professional mental help assistance, the MI approach aids students in recognizing and understanding their need for help.

As a part of the Healthy Minds research project, Eisenberg et al. (2012) reported that one of the strongest correlating factors between intending to seek help and actually seeking help is the student's perception that he or she needs help. An analysis of the Healthy Minds data demonstrates that students who are not receiving treatment most commonly report that they do not seek professional help due to lack of time, preferring to work issues out on their own, and questioning how serious their needs are. Campus leaders with the goals of connecting students to professional help and building resilient campus communities must design their strategies with these barriers in mind.

Conclusion

This chapter explores the relationship between violence and mental health on college campuses. We propose that in addition to all of the important safety and security measures that campuses have implemented recently, a preventative, comprehensive framework needs to be put in place. We outline how an emotionally healthy campus climate promotes help-seeking for those in need before they reach the point of crisis and builds community resilience should a tragedy occur. This proactive approach focuses on the well-being of all students and strives to reduce the stigma of seeking help. To be effective, such a system needs to be comprehensive, connected to campus values and mission, and created by a strategic plan.

Acknowledgments

The authors wish to thank Sara Abelson, senior director of programs for AM, for her generous sharing of expertise and resources. We would also like to thank Hollie McCrea Olson and Connor Haarklau for their assistance.

References

American College Health Association. (2007). National College Health Assessment: Spring 2006 reference group data report (abridged). *Journal of American College Health, 55*(4), 195–206.

American College Health Association. (n.d.). *Healthy campus 2020.* Retrieved from http://www.acha.org/healthycampus

Black, M. C., Basile, K. C., Breiding, M. J., Smith, S. G., Walters, M. L., Merrick, M. T., . . . Stevens, M. R. (2011). *The National Intimate Partner and Sexual Violence Survey (NISVS): 2010 summary report.* Atlanta, GA: National Center for Injury Prevention and Control, Centers for Disease Control and Prevention.

Catalano, S. (2013, November 21). *Intimate partner violence: Attributes of victimization, 1993–2011* (Report No. NCJ 243300). Retrieved from Bureau of Justice Statistics website: http://www.bjs.gov/index.cfm?ty=pbdetail&iid=4801

Centers for Disease Control and Prevention. (2010). *Leading causes of death by age group, all females—United States 2010.* Retrieved from http://www.cdc.gov/women/lcod/2010/WomenAll_2010.pdf

Corrigan, P. W., Druss, B. G., & Perlick, D. A. (2014). The impact of mental illness stigma on seeking and participating in mental health care. *Psychological Science in the Public Interest, 15*(2), 37–70. doi:10.1177/1529100614531398

Curry School of Education. (2012, December 19). *A call for more effective prevention of violence.* Retrieved from http://curry.virginia.edu/articles/sandyhook shooting

Dong, M., Anda, R. F., Felitti, V. J., Dube, S. R., Williamson, D. F., Thompson, C. M., & Giles, W. H. (2004). The interrelatedness of multiple forms of childhood abuse, neglect, and household dysfunction. *Child Abuse & Neglect, 28*(7), 771–784. doi:10.1016/j.chiabu.2004.01.008

Eisenberg, D., Hunt, J., & Speer, N. (2012). Help seeking for mental health on college campuses: Review of evidence and next steps for research and practice. *Harvard Review of Psychiatry, 20*(4), 222–232. doi:10.3109/10673229.2012.712839

Englander, S. (2007). *Understanding violence* (3rd ed.). Mahwah, NJ: Erlbaum.

Fazel, S., & Grann, M. (2006). The population impact of severe mental illness on violent crime. *American Journal of Psychiatry, 163*(8), 1397–1403. doi:10.1176/appi.ajp.163.8.1397

Felitti, V. J., Anda, R. F., Nordenberg, D., Williamson, D. F., Spitz, A. M., Edwards, V., . . . Marks, J. S. (1998). Relationship of childhood abuse and household dysfunction to many of the leading causes of death in adults: The adverse childhood experiences study. *American Journal of Preventive Medicine, 14*(4), 245–258.

Finley, A. (n.d.). *Assessing well-being as a function of learning well.* Retrieved from https://www.aacu.org/sites/default/files/files/CLDE/BTtoPWellbeingInitiative.pdf

Gallagher, R. P. (2006). *National survey of counseling center directors.* Retrieved from http://www.iacsinc.org//home.html

Garske, G. G., & Stewart, J. R. (1999). Stigmatic and mythical thinking: Barriers to vocational rehabilitation services for persons with severe mental illness. *Journal of Rehabilitation, 65*(4), 4–8.

Gatekeeper-trainings at colleges and universities: New findings and next steps for research and practice. (2013). Retrieved from http://healthymindsnetwork.org/research/research-briefs

Grohol, J. M. (2009, October 7). *Online depression screening effective.* Retrieved from http://psychcentral.com/news/2009/10/07/online-depression-screening-effective/8813.html

Guess, A. (2008, March 18). The mental health squeeze. *Inside Higher Ed.* Retrieved from http://www.insidehighered.com/news/2008/03/18/counseling

Keyes, C. (2002). The mental health continuum: From languishing to flourishing in life. *Journal of Health and Social Behavior, 43*(2), 207–222.

Kitzrow, M. A. (2003). The mental health needs of today's college students: Challenges and recommendations. *NASPA Journal, 41*, 167–181.

Kotter, J. P. (2008). *Leading change.* Boston, MA: Harvard Business School Press.

Lipson, S. K. (2014). A comprehensive review of mental health gatekeeper-trainings for adolescents and young adults. *International Journal of Adolescent Medicine and Health, 26*(3), 309–320.

Lipson, S. K., Speer, N., Brunwasser, S., Hahn, E., & Eisenberg, D. (2014). Gatekeeper training and access to mental health care at universities and colleges. *Journal of Adolescent Health, 55*(5), 612–619.

Moskos, M. A., Olson, L., Halbem, S. R., & Gray, D. (2007). Utah youth suicide study: Barriers to mental health treatment for adolescents. *Suicide and Life-Threatening Behavior, 37*(2), 179–186.

Prochaska, J. O., & DiClemente, C. (1983). Stages and processes of self-change of smoking: Toward an integrative model of change. *Journal of Consulting and Clinical Psychology, 51*(3), 390–395.

Reich, J. N. (n.d.). *Connecting the holes to produce a whole: Student well-being as a unifying factor.* Retrieved from http://archive.aacu.org/bringing_theory/index.cfm

Rennison, C. M., & Welchans, S. (2000, May 17). *Intimate partner violence* (Report No. NCJ 178247). Retrieved from Bureau of Justice Statistics website: http://www.bjs.gov/index.cfm?ty=pbdetail&iid=1002

Rosenberg, J. (2014). Mass shootings and mental health policy. *Journal of Sociology & Social Welfare, 41*(1), 107–121.

Simon Fraser University. (n.d.). *Healthy campus community.* Retrieved from https://www.sfu.ca/healthycampuscommunity.html

Steadman, H. J., Mulvey, E. P., Monahan, J., Robins, P. C., Appelbaum, P. S., Grisso, T., . . . Silver, E. (1998). Violence by people discharged from acute psychiatric inpatient facilities and by others in the same neighborhoods. *Archives of General Psychiatry, 55*(5), 393–401. doi:10.1001/archpsyc.55.5.393

Strange, C. C., & Banning, J. H. (2001). *Educating by design: Creating campus learning environments that work.* San Francisco, CA: Jossey-Bass.

Stuart, H. (2003). Violence and mental illness: An overview. *World Psychiatry, 2*(2), 121–124.

U.S. Department of Health and Human Services (HHS) Office of the Surgeon General and National Action Alliance for Suicide Prevention. (2012, September). *2012 National strategy for suicide prevention: Goals and objectives for action.* Washington, DC: HHS.

Whitfield, C. L., Anda, R. F., Dube, S. R., & Felitti, V. J. (2003). Violent childhood experiences and the risk of intimate partner violence in adults: Assessment in a large health maintenance organization. *Journal of Interpersonal Violence, 18*(2), 166–185. doi:10.1177/0886260502238733

Whitlock, J., Wyman, P., & Barreira, P. (2012). *Connectedness & suicide prevention in college settings: Directions and implications for practice.* Retrieved from http://www.selfinjury.bctr.cornell.edu/perch/resources/connectedness-suicide-prevent.pdf

4 Student Development Theory in the Campus Gun Debate

Ainsley Carry and Amy Hecht

Since EDUCATIONAL theorists first offered their psychosocial theories of student development in the 1960s and 1970s, student development theories have provided an important framework for college administrators. Student development theories about identity, masculinity, morality and ethics, and integration have guided practitioners and scholars in their quest to understand young adults and make smarter decisions about supporting their developmental needs. When employed, these theories offer an important perspective on the young-adult mind-set—where students are in their maturation as emerging adults. This is not to suggest that every decision on a college campus must be informed by theory; routine business decisions (e.g., tuition pricing, facilities management, purchasing policies) do not need to be vetted through the lens of students. But decisions that are contingent on behavioral outcomes of college students should be considered through the lens of their development.

The student development theory approach is not foolproof; every theory has its fair share of criticism and bias. Some practitioners debate the efficiency of moving from development theory to practice—the theories do not always translate well in practice. That is, what is written in books and lectured in classrooms does not always work in the field. Another criticism is that some theories were normed on monoethnic and bigender cultures; therefore, broad application is severely limited. The overlapping complexity of each theory, especially because some theories complement each other whereas others contradict each other, is another criticism of the alphabet soup of student development theories.

However, few practitioners would suggest these theories offer no value in the profession. As a guide for decision making, student development theories offer helpful landmarks for examining decisions that assume expectations of students' behavior. Too often decisions that have a direct impact on students have been made without a consideration of how students will respond based on their level of psychosocial development. Practitioner/scholars draw upon student development theories as a natural template for contemplation and discussion about young-adult behavior. They acknowledge that although student development theories all have limitations, the theories at least offer guideposts for deeper considerations about students' behavior.

Through the years, a host of theorists offered thoughtful analysis about how young adults develop and what they are ready for. College administrators used this information to understand how young adults mentally evolve and to determine which interventions they were ready for; the absence of this consideration often lead to intervention failure. College administrators employed these theories to make informed decisions about programs and services. Arthur W. Chickering's theory of identity development (Chickering & Reisser, 1993) describes students' identity development in a series of stages as they go through feeling, thinking, believing, and relating to others; William E. Cross's (1971) model of psychological nigrescence offers a foundation for Black identity development; Lawrence Kohlberg's (1958) stages of moral development suggests that moral reasoning matures in six identifiable stages, explaining how people justify behaviors; and William G. Perry's (1970) theory of intellectual and ethical development proposes that college students pass through a predictable sequence of knowing, from viewing truth in absolute terms of right and wrong to recognizing multiple versions of the truth, each representing legitimate alternatives.

Drawing from the previous observation that student development theories offer important cues about student behavior, the authors contend the debate about college students carrying guns on campus has been void of any rigorous conversation about students' developmental readiness to make this life-altering decision; the decision to arm oneself every day while going to class is no trivial matter. Millions of 18-, 19-, 20-, and 21-year-old undergraduates are expected to contemplate this decision in several states that have approved concealed carry rights in college classrooms and residence halls. The decision to carry a weapon to class has to coincide with the stark realization that one may be forced to use lethal force against a classmate or an intruder. Those who decide not to exercise this new privilege are no better off; they still live, study, dine, and party in environments where the person sitting next to them in class or next door in the residence hall may possess a loaded weapon. The question is: Does that realization change the dynamic of the learning environment enough to stifle learning?

Here, the authors contend the debate has been void of careful analysis through established psychosocial theories that offer perspectives on college students' readiness for important responsibilities. Deciding whether to carry a gun to class, to use that gun in the defense of self or others, and to take the life of a classmate are all life-changing decisions. Police officers and military soldiers train for years in preparation for this responsibility; 18-year-old college students are less likely to have any formal training to prepare them for this sequence of important decisions. Absent from the debate is any intelligent conversation about the intellectual capacity and readiness of college-aged students to make these decisions. The debate has raged on among state and federal governments, largely involving political ideologies, special interest groups, and Second Amendment purists. Both political parties—Democrats and Republicans—stand on opposite sides of the debate, based solely on party lines. Special interest groups, such as the National Rifle Association, stand in opposition of any legislation or discussion that would appear to limit the sale of and access to guns. The motivation driving concealed carry legislation has little to do with students' interests or what is in the best interest of the learning environment.

In this chapter the authors take no sides in the concealed carry on campus debate; the prime objective is to offer an unbiased picture for readers to consider how they might think through this decision when viewing it from a student development perspective, rather than the single-minded political frame (Bolman & Deal, 2013) that dominates the conversation. The discussion is initially considered in terms of Bolman and Deal's work on multiframe thinking—difficult decisions often require multiframe thinking to come to the best solutions. Next the authors acknowledge some of the common arguments for and against concealed carry on campus; there are legitimate arguments on both sides of the issue, but none of these arguments suggest students' level of readiness as a relevant factor in the debate. Finally, the heart of the chapter considers the campus gun debate through Kohlberg's ethical development model. A number of student development theories could be used to continue this conversation, but Kohlberg's work offers the most enlightening perspective.

Multiframe Decision Making

A prerequisite to advancing the gun debate discussion is grappling with the notion of multiframe decision making; this is an effort to bring multiple frames to the debate. There is a widely used optical illusion involving a black-and-white picture of a beautiful, young girl. After viewers get locked into seeing the image of the beautiful girl, they are asked if they can see the image of an unattractive, elderly woman. Looking at the picture from another perspective, some can see the elderly woman; others see the elderly woman first and struggle to see anything else. The same illusion is created with an image of a vase that transforms into two faces facing each other. After seeing the first image, many people struggle to see the other image. Those who eventually see both images realize the lines on either picture never changed; what changed was their mental perspective. Imagine the implications of this type of cognitive shift in organizational decisions. Imagine how many problems present themselves as beautiful opportunities, but are really ill-advised disasters waiting to happen; how many seemingly single-solution problems turn out to have multiple viable solutions. Too often leaders depend upon their initial and narrow perspective in making decisions. They believe their decision is the "best possible," only to later discover alternative possibilities existed.

Few authors make the point about the promise of multiframe thinking better than Bolman and Deal (2013). Bolman and Deal (2013) blamed "cluelessness," which they describe as seeing an incomplete or distorted picture as a result of overlooking or misinterpreting important signals, as the central culprit in management's most significant blunders (p. 5). The failures involving Enron, the *Challenger* space shuttle, and Hurricane Katrina are indicative of managers who were clueless—that is, they failed to consider other perspectives. Decision makers put themselves at a disadvantage when they rely on bad information from advisers, ignore or misinterpret information on their own, or lock themselves into flawed ways of thinking. Luckily, there is a remedy to cluelessness—"reframing." Reframing is "an ability to think about situations in more than one way, which lets you develop alternative diagnoses and strategies" (Bolman & Deal, 2013, p. 5). The idea of reframing is not new; for centuries, critical thinkers have relied on trusted allies to help them see multiple perspectives. The challenge with reframing is being cognizant enough to employ it with every challenge when caught in lifelong patterns of decision-making behavior or forced to make a critical decision in a short period of time or in a crisis.

From this perspective Bolman and Deal (2013) offered *Reframing Organizations* as a solution to the vexing challenge of identifying other frames. They wrote, "A frame is a coherent set of ideas forming a prism or lens that enables you to see and understand more clearly what goes on from day to day" (p. 43). Just like tools, every frame has strengths and weaknesses; no single frame is perfect. "The right tool," they added, "makes a job easier; the wrong one gets in the way. Tools, thus, become useful only when a situation is sized up accurately. . . . Managers who master the hammer and expect all problems to behave like nails find life at work confusing and frustrating" (p. 13). Reframing or multiframe thinking is a powerful tool for adding clarity, generating new options, and considering new angles not previously considered.

Multiframe thinking offers greater effectiveness for decision makers, requires decision makers to move beyond mechanical approaches that dominate complex decision making, and generates multiple layers to apply to the decision. Drawing from sociology, psychology, political science, and anthropology, Bolman and Deal (2013) offered four distinct frames (structural, human resource, political, and symbolic) for leaders to capture a more comprehensive picture:

> The *structural* approach focuses on the architecture of organization—the design of units and subunits, rules and roles, goals and policies. The *human resource* lens emphasizes understanding people—their strengths and foibles, reason and emotion, desire and fears. The *political view* sees organizations as a competitive arena of scarce resources, competing interests, and struggles for power and advantage. Finally, the *symbolic frame* focuses on issues of meaning and faith. It puts ritual, ceremony, story, play, and culture at the heart of organizational life. (pp. 21–22)

Bolman and Deal (2013) continue, saying that:

> A primary cause of managerial failure is faulty thinking rooted in inadequate ideas. Managers and those who try to help them too often rely on narrow models that capture only part of organization life. . . . Learning multiple perspectives, or frames, is a defense against thrashing around without a clue about what you are doing and why. (p. 21)

Multiple frames need to be fully engaged if smart decisions are going to be made about the issue of firearms on campus. The implications are complicated, multidimensional, and emotionally charged; there are no easy answers. For this reason the debate deserves examination from multiple frames. In addition to the structural frames (rules, roles, goals, policies) and political frames (scarce resources, competing interests, power struggles) that have dominated the discussion to this point, this chapter forces readers to strongly consider the human resource or student-development perspective. The student development perspective challenges readers to ponder American college-aged students' strengths, weaknesses, reason, emotions, desires, and fears in light of their new legal authority to carry loaded firearms with them into classrooms, living spaces, libraries, and dining facilities.

The Structural Approach: Federal and State Gun Legislation

The initial perspective employed to tackle difficult problems is typically structural—a look internally to reexamine rules, policies, and procedures that contribute to the problem. Bolman and Deal (2013) suggested the popularity of the structural approach is driven by the fact that

> Rules, policies, standards, and standard operating procedures limit individual discretion and help ensure that behavior is predictable and consistent. Rules and policies govern conditions of work and specify standard ways of completing tasks, handling personnel issues, and relating to customers and other key players in the outer environments. (p. 54)

In other words, the structural perspective and corresponding approach are predictable and safe. They added, "This helps ensure that similar situations are handled in comparable ways. . . . Once a situation is defined as one where a rule applies, the course of action is clear, straightforward, and, in an ideal world, almost automatic" (Bolman & Deal, 2013, pp. 54–55).

The prevailing discourse about guns on campus reflects the assumptions rooted in the structural approach to problem solving—formal rules and standards as a solution to the problem. The hope is that putting rules and structures in place for handling weapons on campus will curb accidents and random acts of violence. The structural approach focuses on analyzing problems through defining relationships. Six assumptions characterize this frame:

1. Organizations exist to achieve established goals and objectives.
2. Organizations increase efficiency and performance through specialization and division of labor.
3. Suitable forms of coordination ensure diverse efforts mesh.
4. Organizations work best when rationality prevails over personal agendas.
5. Structures must be designed to fit an organization's current circumstance.
6. Problems arise and performance suffers from structural deficiencies (Bolman & Deal, 2013, p. 47).

Both federal- and state-level debates about guns in educational environments begin in legislation aimed at structural solutions. In the 1990s a rash of gun violence in schools drew the attention of the federal government. Both the Clinton and Bush administrations presided over legislation aimed at putting structural barriers in place to eliminate gun violence in schools. Two federal acts—the Gun-Free School Zones Act of 1990 (reauthorized in 1996) and the Gun-Free Schools Act of 1994 (reauthorized in 2006)—prohibit guns in areas defined as school zones and recommends minimum sanctions for violators. The Supreme Court (in *United States v. Lopez*) struck down the original version of the law on the grounds that it was not supported by the commerce clause of the Constitution; in 1996 Congress reenacted the Gun-Free School Zones Act, correcting the statute's defects. The revised act included the same prohibitions as the original version. According to these rules, the only people with authorization to carry weapons in a school zone are police officers. The act made it a federal crime to knowingly bring a gun within 1,000 feet of a school or to fire a gun in a school zone and established new standards for behavior in school zones.

The revised Gun-Free Schools Act (1994, 2006) further imposed restrictions on guns in educational environments by focusing on punishment for those found guilty of bringing firearms to school. Federal requirements were imposed on school districts to adopt a policy that required the expulsion for a period of at least 1 year for any student who brought a weapon to a school, a school-sponsored event, or activities on and off school grounds. This way, the act focused on punishment as a tool to restrict gun violence in schools.

Noticing federal legislation of the 1990s was silent with respect to guns on college campuses, state legislators and university governing bodies exercised their authority to establish state laws and internal policies to prohibit or significantly restrict possession of weapons on college campuses. At the time, institutions of higher education either reaffirmed their existing policies or initiated new policies to prohibit guns in university-owned facilities—classrooms, residence halls, athletic facilities, libraries, dining halls, and so on. Similarly, the basic premises of these structural policies were focused on establishing rules, policies, and standards for defining parameters of acceptable behavior and providing standards for taking consistent action against violators.

Everything about early approaches to gun violence began with structure-based solutions. Federal and state legislation defined "school zones," outlined rules and policies, and imposed stiff sanctions on violators. An intense focus on rules, roles, and responsibilities shaped the initial response to gun violence around schools and eventually college campuses. Educational environments exist to achieve stated goals—provide a safe and quality educational experience to students—and these goals are interrupted when weapons that can cause significant bodily harm enter the equation; even the presence of weapons impacts learners' ability to concentrate and focus on learning. For this reason, rules and standards have been the first approach to curbing gun violence.

Campus Shootings and Emergence of the Political Perspective

After campus shootings at Virginia Tech in 2007 and Northern Illinois University in 2008, and the election of U.S. President Barack Obama, a Democrat, the tenor of the campus gun debate shifted perspectives from structural to political. After decades of near universal agreement among Democrats and Republicans on the need to keep guns out of educational environments, a new cry to repeal federal and state laws prohibiting guns in educational environments emerged. Minimal challenges were aimed at the Gun-Free School Zones Act of 1990, passed by Congress and upheld by the Supreme Court. Instead, colleges' and universities' campus policies prohibiting guns on campus were attacked. Legislators proposed legislation to strike down university policies that prohibited guns on campus; advocates called for college students and faculty to carry concealed weapons to defend against attacks. The states that reversed and those that maintained their positions were uniformly divided based on political alignment. Predominantly Republican states favored efforts to permit guns on campus, whereas Democratic states fought against allowing guns on campus. The issue is almost entirely viewed according to a political frame.

The *political frame*, as defined by Bolman and Deal (2013) in their work *Reframing Organizations*, more accurately describes the composition of the argument today. Advocates for detractors from guns in schools are divided by interest groups; they have enduring differences, and stakeholders are focused on their personal interest. This is consistent with the five propositions that make up Bolman and Deal's (2013) political frame:

1. Organizations are coalitions of assorted individuals and interest groups.
2. Coalition members have enduring differences in values, beliefs, information, interests, and perceptions of reality.
3. Most important decisions involve allocating scarce resources—who gets what.
4. Scarce resources and enduring differences put conflict at the center of day-to-day dynamics and make power the most important asset.
5. Goals and decisions emerge from bargaining and negotiating among competing stakeholders jockeying for their own interests. (pp. 194–195)

Bolman and Deal's (2013) political frame succinctly captures the perspective around the conversation. Opponents on both sides of the debate, "coalitions of assorted individuals and interest groups" (p. 194), pivot their position based on political, rather than structural, arguments. The gun debate is overwhelmingly influenced on both sides by lobbyists and special interest groups that have competing interests. Opponents "have enduring differences in values, beliefs, information, interest, and perceptions of reality" (p. 195). The differences in values and beliefs between the two parties—Democratic and Republican—are rarely more divided than they are in regard to this topic. And these enduring differences "put conflict at the center of day-to-day dynamics and make power the most important asset" (p. 196). Rather than having reasonable discussions about practical tools to eliminate gun violence on campus, "competing stakeholders [are] jockeying for their own interests" (p. 196). The debate about guns on campus is wrapped in a political context, and therefore reasonable dialogue on both sides—in favor and against—is hampered by interest groups, enduring differences, and power struggles. Nothing defines the gun debate better than competition for personal interests; consequently, the developmental needs and personal interest of those impacted the most—college students—are practically ignored.

In defining the political perspective, Bolman and Deal (2013) also identified important relationships among politics, divergent interests, scarce resources, conflict, and power. The campus gun debate has become a political football. Greater interest is invested in special interests, and losers (Democrats or Republicans) of the debate fear the loss of political power. Bolman and Deal wrote, "Politics is the realistic process of making decisions and allocating resources in a context of scarcity and divergent interests" (2013, p. 190). Under these conditions conflict inevitably emerges. Further, they wrote,

> The political frame stresses that the combination of scarce resources and divergent interests produces conflict. . . . Interest groups vie for policy concessions. If one group controls the policy process, others may be frozen out. . . . The political prism puts more emphasis on strategy and tactics than on resolution of conflict. (p. 206)

Whereas the 1990s saw bipartisan agreement on structural limits on guns in school zones, since 2008 the matter has divided along party lines. Where there was once little disagreement among state legislators that firearms had no place in educational environments from kindergarten through college, in 2014 states were almost equally divided on this topic. In the 1990s, federal and state legislators reacted to threats of gun violence in educational environments by implementing tough federal legislation, which defined parameters and provided guidelines for minimum sanctions—a structural frame solution. By 2008, the reaction to gun violence in educational environments had shifted to a political tug-of-war.

Advocates for Guns on Campus

Advocates for guns on campus root their position in the Second Amendment to the U.S. Constitution: "A well regulated Militia, being necessary to the security of a free State, the right of the people to keep and bear Arms, shall not be infringed." It has frequently been debated whether the Second Amendment applied exclusively to regulated militias and protection of states. In 2008, the Supreme Court (*District of Columbia v. Heller*) definitively held that the Second Amendment protects an *individual's* right to possess a firearm unconnected with service in a militia and to use that weapon for traditionally lawful purposes, such as self-defense. From this perspective, advocates deemed it a violation of one's constitutional rights for institutions of higher education to prohibit students from carrying guns on campus. They further argued that armed faculty and students would be better able to defend themselves from someone with a gun. Furthermore, law-abiding citizens are vulnerable in gun-free zones where individuals intending to do harm can do so unopposed. Their solution is to arm faculty and students in an effort to assist law enforcement officers responding to classroom shooters.

As of 2014, seven states repealed firearm prohibitions on college campuses: Colorado, Idaho, Kansas, Mississippi, Oregon, Utah, and Wisconsin. Institutions of higher education in these states cannot make policies that restrict students from bringing weapons to campus (Law Center to Prevent Gun Violence, 2014). Legislators in these states successfully argued that allowing students to defend themselves would reduce, rather than increase, on-campus gun violence (Utah); established a state statute specifically naming public colleges as "public entities" (Utah Code Ann. § 76-10-500(2), 1999) that do not have the authority to ban concealed carry (Utah); and proposed that only the legislature can regulate the use, sale, and possession of firearms, and therefore college campuses overstep their boundaries when dictating concealed carry rights (Colorado and Oregon).

Yet in some states, institutions managed to carve out a few exceptions still allowing them to limit firearms on campus. In Kansas, guns are not permitted in buildings that have "adequate security measures" (Kansas, 2013). Wisconsin institutions lobbied to limit firearms where signs are posted at every entrance explicitly stating that weapons are prohibited. In Mississippi, college administrators managed to limit weapons to those who have taken a voluntary course on safe handling and use of firearms by a certified instructor. Although seemingly minor limitations, they are likely to moderate the influx of weapons that could potentially enter classrooms and residence halls.

Opponents of Guns on Campus

Arguments against firearms on campus are equally persuasive. Those opposed to firearms on campus express concern about how the presence of weapons may impact the feeling of the learning environment. They believe it would inhibit dialogue by making students and faculty feel less safe to freely debate ideas in class and severely distract from the learning environment when students know their classmates are armed. They are concerned that college students' accidental mishandling of firearms in public spaces—classrooms, residence halls, fraternity houses, libraries—has a high probability of causing serious injuries or death. They caution that colleges are emotionally volatile environments where faculty and staff at times must deliver bad news (e.g., failing grades, disciplinary decisions, dismissal from a program or an organization, failure to qualify for a scholarship) to students. Some professors might be afraid to issue poor grades if they fear a student may be carrying a gun. Discipline officers may live in constant fear that their decision to suspend or expel a student could result in retaliation.

A growing category of concern is related to students' mental health and readiness to handle the responsibility of carrying a firearm. Rates of mental illness (U.S. Department of Health and Human Services, 2002), suicide (American College Health Association, 2009; Miller & Hemenway, 2001), and alcohol abuse (Siebel, 2008) are high among young adults between the ages of 18 and 25. In a 2011 study, between 9% and 11% of college students seriously considered suicide in the previous school year, and about 1,100 college students commit suicide each year (Hirsch, Web, & Jeglic, 2011). When a gun enters this mix, a suicide attempt becomes considerably more lethal, as 85% of gun suicide attempts are fatal (Vyrostek, Annest, & Ryan, 2004). There is concern that increased access to firearms, whether their own or their roommates', could increase the fatality of suicide attempts.

Alcohol and drug use in college further complicates the issue. The college years are a period when young adults are testing their limits with alcohol, and some are experimenting with illegal drugs for the first time. Accidents (e.g., car accidents; falls down stairwells; and unanticipated, unintended outcomes of high-risk games) are commonly associated with overconsumption of alcohol. Hallucinations and paranoia induced by drug use are concerns when guns are readily available. Alcohol and drugs increase the risk of injury for students in environments where guns are present. Alcohol is involved in approximately 66% of college student suicides, 95% of violent crime on campus, and 90% of campus rapes (Miller, Hemenway, & Wechsler, 2002). Institutions are working to address these issues, but they are not going away anytime soon. Many higher education administrators argue that adding weapons into this situation only exacerbates the problem and is likely to have deadly consequences.

Colleges and universities have created teams to help manage information on students of concern. This can include students who are a risk to self as well as students with behavioral issues. These teams rely on a number of administrators to process information and respond in a timely and appropriate manner. There is concern that collaborative efforts to keep campus communities safe would be further complicated with firearms added into the equation.

From a mental readiness perspective, neurologists argue that the human brain is not fully developed until the early 20s. The last portion of the brain to be developed is the one that controls impulses and the ability to plan ahead, two signs of mature adulthood. Until the brain is fully developed, individuals are more susceptible to risk-taking behaviors (Steinberg, 2007); because of the predilection for risk taking, the introduction of guns to an environment largely composed of college-aged people could lead to serious or even deadly consequences. In a study conducted by Miller et al. (2002), students who reported having a gun on campus disproportionately engaged in high-risk behaviors endangering themselves and others. The study concluded that guns did not lead to a safer or more secure campus. Instead, those individuals with guns contributed to a more dangerous environment.

The International Association of Campus Law Enforcement Administrators (IACLEA) (www.iaclea.org) argues against students and faculty carrying weapons on campus as a defense mechanism against campus shooters. It questions how first responders can adequately tell the difference between armed civilians and armed assailants. In an active shooter scenario, a student or faculty member with a gun would only distract law enforcement from identifying the true perpetrator, injure innocent students, and possibly get injured or killed by a police officer who suspects the student or faculty member of being the campus shooter.

Although legislation has been codified in some states, others are split on the issue of banning or permitting concealed weapons on college campuses. Currently, 21 states continue their ban on carrying a concealed weapon on college campuses: California, Florida, Georgia, Illinois, Louisiana, Massachusetts, Michigan, Missouri, Nebraska, Nevada, New Jersey, New Mexico, New York, North Carolina, North Dakota, Ohio, Oklahoma, South Carolina, Tennessee, Texas, and Wyoming. The remaining 22 states leave the decision to the college or university administration: Alabama, Alaska, Arizona, Arkansas, Connecticut, Delaware, Hawaii, Indiana, Iowa, Kentucky, Maine, Maryland, Minnesota, Montana, New Hampshire, Pennsylvania, Rhode Island, South Dakota, Vermont, Virginia, Washington, and West Virginia (Law Center to Prevent Gun Violence, 2014).

Student Development

The central tenet of this chapter is the thoughtful inclusion of the human resource or student development perspective in the on-campus gun debate. Students' maturity to live on a college campus with access to firearms, their capacity to make life-and-death decisions about when it is appropriate to use lethal force, and their ability to deal with the psychological aftermath of accidentally injuring or seeing a classmate killed by a gun are important developmental considerations for administrators. The prevailing debate has centered on structural and political arguments to the detriment of critical discussions about the emotional and psychological capacity required to contemplate the use of deadly force to resolve threats in the classroom. How these circumstances impact students' ongoing development and ability to learn is important. There is perhaps no greater emotional decision than that which involves potentially taking the life of another person.

Consider the complexities of the scenario faced by 18-year-old college students on campuses that allow concealed carry. At 8:00 a.m. a college freshman living in a residence hall is packing his backpack for class. In the backpack he inserts textbooks, notebooks, pens, and a calculator for math class. Today he has three classes—one auditorium-sized class and two small classes with fewer than 25 classmates. In between classes, he has a group meeting in the library, and then plans to go to lunch with friends at a local diner. He opens his dresser drawer where his handgun is stored. Every morning he decides whether to pack the handgun. A series of questions run through his mind at an unconscious level: Do I feel threatened today? Is today the day a shooter will visit one of my classes? Will my classmates have their guns today? Are the places that I plan to go today—classroom, library, dining hall, math lab—appropriate for a loaded handgun? Is my gun safely stored in my backpack so that it will not accidently discharge and injure or kill a classmate? Will I be able to decipher between a life-threatening danger and a scary moment? Am I prepared to take someone's life to defend myself? He decides to pack a firearm in his backpack for the day. The day goes without any need to defend himself with a gun. Tomorrow he has to go through the decision-making process again.

Kohlberg's Theory of Moral Development

Kohlberg's theory of moral development suggests that moral reasoning is the foundation of ethical behavior (1958). The general hypothesis is that people's behaviors become increasingly ethical, consistent, and refined as they mature and advance to higher stages of development. That is, things that were acceptable in youth become less acceptable as one grows older and, theoretically, people become more morally conscious. In Kohlberg's theory, each stage addresses how people justify ethical or unethical behavior, and moral development is a lifelong process. Kohlberg's theory includes three levels and six stages.

On level one, the preconventional level, the morality of one's actions is based on their consequences; what is right or wrong is completely dependent on external consequences (e.g., punishment). The preconventional level is further defined by two stages. In stage one, obedience and punishment, action is perceived as morally wrong only when it is followed by punishment. The severity of the punishment indicates how bad the behavior is considered, and deference is given to superior power. In stage two, self-interest, behavior is morally right or wrong depending on what is in the best interest of the individual absent relationships to other groups of people. Interest in the needs of others is limited to the point where it might further one's own interests.

On level two, the conventional level, moral reasoning involves judging the morality of actions by comparing them to the views and expectations of society. At this level individuals rigidly adhere to rules and follow society's norms even when there are no consequences. What is moral is predominantly controlled by things outside self. The appropriateness or fairness of rules is seldom questioned. Two stages further describe the conventional level. In stage three, interpersonal accord and conformity, individuals are influenced by approval or disapproval from others. They try to live up to society's expectations and be a "good boy" or "good girl." Their motivation to behave is based only in their interest to further support their perceived social roles. In stage four, authority and social order obedience, individuals obey laws and social norms because of their importance in maintaining an orderly society. They sense an obligation to uphold the law because it protects the rights of all. Therefore, violating the law becomes morally wrong.

On level three, the postconventional level, there is a realization that an individual's morality can be separate and different from society's. The individual's own perspective takes primacy over society's view; therefore, individuals at this level may not have to follow rules that are misaligned with their own values. People who exhibit postconventional morality live by their own ethical principles and view rules as changeable, not as absolute dictates that must be obeyed without question. This level is also further defined by two stages. In stage five, social contract, laws are viewed as social contracts rather than rigid edicts, and laws that do not promote the general welfare should be changed. Each person has the right to his or her unique opinions, rights, and values. In stage six, universal ethical principles, moral reasoning is based on abstract reasoning using universal ethical principles. Laws are valid as long as they are grounded in a commitment to justice. This involves an individual imagining what he or she would do in another's shoes if the individual believed what another person imagines to be true. The individual takes action because it is right, not because it avoids punishment, is in his or her best interest, is expected by others, is legal, or is previously agreed upon.

Kohlberg's Theory and Guns on Campus

Kohlberg's theory inspires consideration of the fact that college-aged students are evolving adults at various stages of moral development. On a campus of hundreds or thousands of students, students are likely present at every level of moral development. Preconventional thinkers focus on self-interest and avoidance of punishment. As such, in weighing the decision to pack a firearm and possibly use it on campus, the preconventional thinker has a moral disposition aimed toward preservation of self-interest absent relationships with other group members. How would this disposition play out in the face of an active shooter situation? Police officers take a pledge and are trained to serve and protect others before protecting themselves. Absent appropriate training, the preconventional thinker may be as dangerous a threat to others as an active shooter intentionally trying to do harm.

On the other hand, students who are conventional thinkers are focused on obeying society's norms without question. These students will approach the decision to carry a firearm into class or a residence hall much differently from their preconventional-minded peers. On campuses where firearms are permitted, conventional thinkers may be tormented by the dichotomy between campus rules, which permit firearms on campus, and societal norms, which constantly send messages about the dangers of firearms. Although it is legal for most people to own and possess a firearm, the contradiction of this societal norm with campus culture will pose an emotional tug-of-war for conventional thinkers. They will struggle with the realization that they are at a disadvantage in environments where others freely carry firearms in the classroom and living spaces. In an effort to level the playing field or to fit in, they may uncomfortably arm themselves and become an accident waiting to happen. This daily realization may cause stress and hamper learning. Students from universities in Texas and Washington recently were surveyed about allowing concealed firearms on campus. According to research led by Jeffrey Bouffard at Sam Houston State University's College of Criminal Justice, more students were uncomfortable with concealed weapons on campus than were at ease with guns on college grounds (Cavanaugh, Bouffard, Wells, & Nobles, 2012).

For postconventional thinkers, there is more separation between their moral compass and society; they do not feel compelled to agree with what is believed by society in general. This group of thinkers may be more at ease with the idea that some classmates may be armed in class; they will not be judgmental toward those who decide either way. In the same vein, postconventional thinkers will not experience the dissonance, unlike their conventional-thinking peers, if they themselves decide to exercise their rights to bear arms. They realize their moral character will remain intact regardless of their decision to carry a firearm and how society in general may perceive this decision. Postconventional thinkers differing from their preconventional peers, will not arm themselves purely based on self-interest; they are more likely to take this position in an effort to protect the social contract—the unwritten agreement among a campus community to protect each other.

Conclusion

The nation is struggling with a formidable challenge—how best to curtail mass shootings in educational environments. Mass shootings at Columbine, Virginia Tech, Northern Illinois, and Sandy Hook are grim reminders of the lethal power of firearms in educational settings. The challenge has forced the nation to examine the ugly truth about our gun culture; in well-intended efforts to uphold the Second Amendment of the Constitution we have seen the unintended consequences of wide availability of firearms. At one extreme, advocates suggest implementing measures to severely restrict access to firearms; at the other extreme, advocates propose lifting prohibitions on firearms in educational environments as a self-defense measure. Neither side is likely to prevail, and the answer is perhaps somewhere in the middle.

The prevailing approach to gun violence in educational environments has been through structural actions (rules, laws, policies, sanctions) and political actions (power, control, special interests groups). Gun laws such as the Gun-Free School Zones Act (1990, 1996) and Gun-Free Schools Act (1994, 2006) drew bipartisan support to create structural guidelines around firearm restrictions and punishment in educational environments. Since 2008, the political tug-of-war about firearms in educational environments has introduced an additional perspective to the argument. These perspectives, structural and political, are essential to the argument and have value; both broaden the scope of solutions and force advocates on both sides to carefully consider other perspectives. Neither position should be ignored or disregarded; instead, rigorous consideration is required.

However, the prevailing perspectives unveiled only two dimensions of this multidimensional challenge. Bolman and Deal (2013), authors of *Reframing Organizations*, reminded us that multiframe decision making is the antidote to cluelessness. The authors offered a model to view complicated problems in organizations through four perspectives—structural, political, human resource, and symbolic. In this chapter, we apply multiframe thinking to the firearm debate. We insert a student development (human resource) perspective into the firearms on campus debate. Kohlberg's theory of moral development offers a meaningful perspective for us to ponder the spectrum of student moral dispositions. Restricting or expanding firearm access in an educational environment has important implications based on students' level of moral reasoning. Students' mind-sets at each level—preconventional, conventional, and postconventional—have meaningful implications. Ignoring these developmental stages is negligent, whereas studying them could provide important clues as to how college-aged students may respond.

References

American College Health Association. (2009). American College Health Association National College Health Assessment spring 2008 reference group data report (abridged). *Journal of American College Health, 56*(5), 447–488.

Bolman, L. G., & Deal, T. E. (2013). *Reframing organizations: Artistry, choice, and leadership* (5th ed.). San Francisco, CA: Jossey-Bass.

Cavanaugh, M. R., Bouffard, J. A., Wells, W., & Nobles, N. R. (2012). Student attitudes toward concealed handguns on campus at 2 universities. *American Journal of Public Health, 102*(12), 2245–2247.

Chickering, A. W., & Reisser, L. (1993). *Education and identity* (2nd ed.). San Francisco, CA: Jossey-Bass.

Cross, W. E. (1971). The Negro-to-Black conversion experience. *Black World, 10*(9), 13–27.

District of Columbia v. Heller, 554 U.S. 570 (2008).

Gun-Free Schools Act of 1994, 20 U.S.C. §§ 7151 et seq (1994).

Hirsch, J. K., Web, J. R., & Jeglic, E. L. (2011). Forgiveness, depression, and suicidal behavior among a diverse sample of college students. *Clinical Psychology, 67*(1), 896–906.

Kansas, H.B. 2052, 85th Leg., Reg. Sess. (2013).

Kohlberg, L. (1958). *The development of modes of thinking and choices in years 10 to 16* (Unpublished doctoral dissertation). University of Chicago.

Law Center to Prevent Gun Violence. (November 1, 2013). *Guns in schools policy summary.* Retrieved from http://smartgunlaws.org/guns-in-schools-policy-summary/

Miller, M., Hemenway, D. (2001). Gun prevalence and the risk of suicide: A review. *Harvard Health Policy Review. 2*(2), 29–37.

Miller, M., Hemenway, D., & Wechsler, H. (2002). Guns and gun threats at college. *Journal of American College Health, 5*(12), 57–65.

Perry G., Jr. (1970). *Forms of intellectual and ethical development in the college years: A scheme.* New York, NY: Holt, Rinehart, and Winston.

Siebel, B. The case against guns on campus. *George Mason University Civil Rights Law Journal. 18*(2), 319–337.

Steinberg, L. (2007). Risk taking in adolescence: New perspectives from brain and behavioral science. *Current Directions in Psychological Science, 16*(2), 55–59.

U.S. Constitution, Second Amendment. (1791).

U.S. Department of Health and Human Services. (2002) *National survey on drug use and health.* Retrieved from http://www.samhsa.gov/data/node/20

Utah Code Ann. § 76-10-500(2) (1999).

Vyrostek, S. B., Annest, J. L., & Ryan, G. W. (2004). *Surveillance for fatal and nonfatal injuries—United States 2001.* Retrieved from http://www.cdc.gov/mmwr/preview/mmwrhtml/ss5307a1.htm

5 Risk and Threat Assessment

John H. Dunkle and Brian J. Mistler

IN THE aftermath of mass shootings on college campuses over the past several years, institutions of higher education
(IHEs) in the United States have moved to implement violence prevention measures like no other time in history. Although campus
threat assessment teams have existed on some campuses for quite
some time, they have recently become increasingly commonplace
(Brunner, Wallace, Reymann, Sellers, & McCabe, in press). In fact,
two states, Virginia and Illinois, are the first to have passed laws
that require all IHEs to have violence prevention programs, including campus threat assessment teams, to help detect, intervene with,
and monitor individuals who may pose a danger to campuses. The
purpose of this chapter is to provide an overview of risk/threat assessment and its role in preventing gun violence on campuses. We begin
by defining *risk/threat assessment*, followed by a review of risk/threat
assessment team frameworks and critical issues/questions for campuses to address in developing and implementing a team. Next, we
address the roles and responsibilities various members may play on
risk/threat assessment teams. Finally, we discuss the advantages of a
communitywide approach to reducing violence on campuses. Risk/
threat assessment teams can and must do a great deal, but IHEs cannot rely on only the team members for preventing violence. Campus
community members play a critical role in creating a broad safety
net, and we discuss some of the important areas of training in both
recognizing and reporting potential threats that are useful for college
campuses. The authors would like to state up front that we understand campuses vary widely in terms of size of institution, private
versus public, rural versus urban, and the resources they possess.
Therefore, we want to be clear that the issues we discuss in this
chapter may not be rel evant to or possible for all campuses.

What Is Risk/Threat Assessment?

Historical Context

In the aftermath of the tragic gun violence on the campus of Virginia Polytechnic Institute and State University (hereafter Virginia Tech) in April 2007, the U.S. Secret Service, the U.S. Department of Education, and the Federal Bureau of Investigation launched a collaborative effort to explore violence on college and university campuses and how such tragedies could be prevented in the future. The team charged with undertaking the effort published its findings and recommendations in a final report (Drysdale, Modzeleski, & Simons, 2010). A major focus of the research effort was to examine the scope of the problem of targeted campus violence. Between 1900 and 2008, the researchers found, through review of public documentation, that 272 incidents of targeted violence occurred on or near IHE campuses, with almost 60% of the documented incidents occurring in the past 20–30 years. (The investigators urged readers to use caution in making unduly broad conclusions, because relying on the public reports often resulted in limited information gathering, especially with the incidents from the earlier part of the century.) In many ways, the 2010 initiative replicated a similar study of primary and secondary education settings conducted by the U.S. Department of Education and the U.S. Secret Service, entitled the *Safe School Initiative* (Vossekuil, Fein, Reddy, Borum, & Modzeleski, 2004). This study was initiated after the horrific shootings at Columbine High School in Colorado in April 1999. Investigating a more limited time period, Vossekuil et al. (2004) researched the scope of the problem in primary and secondary school settings and reported that between 1974 and 2000 there were 37 incidents of targeted violence in schools.

The other major finding from both studies was that in most of the incidents the violence was premeditated, and the perpetrators demonstrated behaviors and/or communicated information to others that indicated that they were on a pathway toward violence. However, those who observed the behaviors or received the communications seldom knew if, or where, they could/should share information, and, therefore, the unfortunate outcome was that there was no intervention to prevent the violence. These key findings pointed to the obvious conclusion that potential violence can be prevented with careful evaluation of available information about persons expressing violent intention via verbal/written communications or other behaviors. Therefore, the investigators concluded that threat assessment strategies are the most promising violence prevention strategies for schools and IHEs.

Risk/Threat Assessment Defined

The aforementioned reports defined *threat assessment* as a fact-based investigative and analytical process, formally evaluating behaviors and communications and the degree and nature of a threat in relationship to a specific target, with the intent of stopping an act of violence before it occurs. It is important to understand the historical differences between "risk assessment" and "threat assessment." Risk assessment models tend to focus on the risk of a particular individual to commit acts of violence. These approaches have looked at dangerousness prediction, have understood violence risk as intrinsic to a person, and have assumed that violence risk is stable over time (implicit) and that the goal is accuracy of assessment of a person. More recently, in the field of assessment as a whole, approaches have evolved to a violence threat/risk assessment. This approach understands violence risk as a function of the threat presented by a particular person *in a particular context*, and sees violence risk as dynamic and varied, requiring iterative approaches to assessment and monitoring, with an ultimate goal of dual threat/risk management.

This move also precipitated a shift from the initial emphasis on clinical interviews, intuitive risk factors in which clinical opinion formation was often unstructured (or structure was not explicitly articulated), and risk communication offered in dichotomous terms to a more broad-based, context-informed, methodical, and scientifically informed approach. Thus, current leading approaches to threat assessment include clinical interviews as only one of many data sources. They also place an emphasis on research-supported risk factors and clinical judgment that tend to be more structured and linked explicitly to data, leading to risk communication offered in probabilistic terms (Day Shaw, Mistler, & Book, 2013).

Indeed, an objective and fact-based process is a critical one for threat assessment. Threat assessment that is based on hearsay, misconceptions, misinformation, and/or stereotypes is problematic and potentially dangerous for the campus community. For instance, institutions that take an adverse action against a student based on known or perceived mental health issues could violate disability laws. The U.S. Department of Education's Office for Civil Rights (OCR) is the federal agency with explicit authority for enforcement of various federal laws, including, but not limited to, Title II of the Americans with Disabilities Act (ADA) of 1990 and Section 504 of the Rehabilitation Act of 1973. These laws prohibit discrimination based on a known or perceived disability, including mental health disabilities. The OCR has emphasized the importance of an objective and individualized process tailored to the specific student of concern, in order to determine if the student meets criteria of a "direct threat standard." In a letter summarizing an investigation of a student complaint brought against Spring Arbor University, the OCR defined the *direct threat standard* and the individualized and objective process that a college or university must undertake when assessing a student who may pose a threat to the community. This quotation comes directly from the letter:

> The "direct threat" standard applies to situations where a university proposes to take adverse action against a student, whose disability poses significant risk to the health or safety of others. A significant risk constitutes a high probability of substantial harm and not just a slightly increased speculative or remote risk. In determining whether a student poses a direct threat, the university must make an individualized assessment, based on a reasonable judgment that relies on current medical knowledge or on the best available objective evidence, to ascertain: the nature, duration, and severity of the risk; the probability that the potential injury will actually occur; and whether reasonable modifications of policies, practices, or procedures will sufficiently mitigate the risk. (OCR Letter to Spring Arbor University, 2010, p. 9)

Students, however, are not the only potential group of individuals who may pose a threat of violence to a campus. Faculty, staff, and individuals not directly affiliated with the institution may also be potential perpetrators of violence and require assessment and intervention. In cases involving faculty and staff, consultation with human resources and legal counsel with expertise in employment laws will be necessary to ensure that a nondiscriminatory and fair threat assessment process occurs. For individuals not affiliated with the university, campus officials may need to coordinate with local, off-campus, or other authorities to ensure the safety of the campus community.

Threat Assessment Process

Once a formal threat assessment inquiry has begun, there are various elements to the process and key questions that may be considered. We address some of the major questions and issues here, as room does not allow for an in-depth discussion of all the nuances and issues to consider. Deisinger, Randazzo, O'Neill, and Savage (2008) offered a threat assessment flowchart that provides a general overview of key decision points in threat assessment. When the campus is made aware of a person who may pose a threat to the community, the first order of business in the threat assessment process is to decide whether the situation is imminent, requiring immediate intervention by law enforcement. Of course, there must be agreement about what constitutes an imminent situation. In many cases, an imminent situation involves an individual with access to a weapon expressing intention to do harm to at least one person.

If an imminent situation does not exist, other information needs to be collected to determine the level of risk that a person may pose to the campus community. Campus threat assessment teams (see this chapter's discussion on team frameworks) must begin the process of collecting as much information as possible about the individual of concern. The team needs to determine first what the individual's relationship is vis-à-vis the campus. Is the individual a student, faculty/staff member, or nonaffiliated other person? Answering this question will aid in accessing the appropriate team (should multiple campus teams exist), and in determining what resources need to be accessed on and off campus.

Once the individual's status has been verified (or concurrent with efforts to do so, if the situation appears more time critical), the campus team begins to gather information to assist in determining the threat level. Information may come from a variety of sources. For example, it is important to initiate discussions with collateral parties who have observed the individual engaging in concerning behavior. It is critical to ensure that collateral parties be encouraged to report observations and specific behaviors instead of only conjectures or fears. Other information can be gathered from searching public profiles of the individual on social media, which at the time of publication includes Facebook, Instagram, Twitter, blogs, YouTube, Yik Yak, and other sites. In fact, simply doing a general query via any search engine, such as Google, may be beneficial to ensure a comprehensive online inquiry. In addition, teams may review e-mails and other correspondences that an individual may have posted or sent. Although social media and electronic correspondences are good sources of data, one must use caution in coming to conclusions based only on these sources. Electronic information can be easily misinterpreted, but it can serve as one source of data for the team to use in the broader assessment process.

Another source of information in cases involving students is a review of disciplinary records. In addition, the team may want to consult with the student's academic program to determine academic progress and attendance history. Often, struggles in academic areas and attendance inconsistencies are indicators that a student may be in distress or perhaps worse. The campus team may determine that parental/emergency contact is the most appropriate step; therefore, the dean of students or other conduct officer can consult parental/emergency notification policies for the institution. A similar source of information can be accessed in cases involving faculty/staff. Campus teams may consult with their human resource departments to determine if an employee has a documented record of concerning behavior. Most campuses regularly do background checks prior to hiring employees; therefore, the results of the background check may be a useful source of information. With all potential perpetrators, campus law enforcement may access criminal history records. This process may involve contacting other local, state, and federal authorities.

Teams may also consider utilizing a variety of objective measures that have been developed to assess risk/threat. However, we caution that the measures should not be relied on solely for determining risk/threat; rather they should be adjuncts to other gathered information and team judgment. For example, although a student may score low on a self-reported measure of violence, if team members are aware of specific threats or trained mental health staff report concerns based on clinical interviews or professional judgment, safety should not be assumed and further assessment or action may be required. Equally, if a student reports high levels of hostility or otherwise triggers concern based on a standardized instrument, but there have been no specific threats, monitoring should begin or continue at an elevated level to increase the likelihood of early detection should the risk level increase. Also, if a team is going to utilize risk/threat assessment instruments, team members should be trained in their administration and interpretation. Some example measures include the Workplace Assessment of Violence Risk (WAVR-21; Meloy, White, & Hart, 2013) and Classification of Violence Risk (COVR; Monahan et al., 2006).

On some occasions, a campus threat assessment team may want to enlist the services of professionals who conduct forensic and fitness-for-duty evaluations when questions arise around an individual's ability to perform in the academic setting or at work. These evaluations can be quite costly and require highly specialized and trained psychologists or psychiatrists to conduct them. Forensic and fitness-for-duty evaluations typically involve extensive interviewing, collateral information gathering, and formal psychological testing using various measures. They can involve several days of meeting with the individual being evaluated. The results of these extensive evaluations can offer campus teams a great deal of information, including critical information around risk for violence. These types of evaluations also help campus team members to make decisions about fitness to return to academic programs and/or work. Although these evaluations are costly, it is in the best interest of the institution to choose a professional to carry out the evaluation and to pay for its completion. In this way, the institution is the "client" and the assessor is looking out for the interest of the campus and the community. The alternative would be to have the individual of concern locate and pay for the evaluation. However, with this approach, the evaluator would be advocating for the individual, and the individual may choose an evaluator who does not have the competency to conduct these types of evaluations. During an important and time-sensitive threat assessment process is a less-than-ideal time to be searching for a well-qualified forensic psychologist; therefore, developing a relationship with one or more professionals, including agreement on pricing and internal budget approvals, is suggested as a routine activity in advance of any crisis.

Through careful review of the various sources of information, threat assessment team members are able to evaluate behaviors, ask critical questions, and review other data to determine if an individual is on a pathway toward violence. The more concerning behaviors that are present, the higher the likelihood that the individual may be on a pathway toward violence and be a higher threat to the campus community. One of the first areas to assess is whether the individual of concern has explicitly expressed a desire/intent to harm another person. It is also important to evaluate whether the individual has committed violent acts in the past, as past behaviors are often predictive of future behaviors. Further, the more closely related the past behaviors are to the target behaviors (violence, in this case) the more likely they are to be predictive. Violent acts could have been committed against self, others, and/or inanimate objects. Clarifying whether the person of concern has access to and/or possesses a weapon, such as a gun, knife, or chemical, is also a critical task for the team. A great deal of research has pointed to the conclusion that restricting an individual's access to the means for committing violence significantly reduces the likelihood that a violent outcome will occur (Bryan, Stone, & Rudd, 2011).

Individuals who express intent to commit violence or actually proceed to commit a violent act often feel wronged by others and have accumulated a list of grievances (Meloy, 2006). These individuals are colloquially referred to as "grievance collectors." For instance, an individual may have experienced the breakup of a romantic relationship, a poor work performance review, and a recent arrest for driving while under the influence. In combination with other risk factors, the accumulation of grievances becomes a warning sign for potential violence. Somewhat related to grievance collecting is the act of stalking and its relationship to potential violence. Stalking behavior is the unwanted, and perhaps intimidating, active pursuit of another individual. The behavior may be accompanied by an acute psychotic process known as erotomanic delusions (Meloy, 2006). These delusions involve, even in the presence of substantial evidence to the contrary, the stalker's firm belief that the love object reciprocates the romantic feelings. The stalker becomes even more persistent and may eventually commit a crime of violence when the feelings are unrequited. A notorious example of these behaviors was the Virginia Tech senior, Seung-Hui Cho, who killed 32 people and injured 17 others in a shooting rampage in April 2007. Cho reportedly engaged in stalking behavior with two women and vented many of his grievances on video prior to the acts of violence.

Levels of Risk, Action Plans, and Monitoring

Upon completion of the threat assessment process described earlier, the team must assign a level of risk, on a continuum of no risk to severe/high risk, and put a plan into action. Certainly, campuses can come up with their own levels of risk. However, Deisinger et al. (2008) provided excellent sample priority levels for threat cases in their handbook.

Campus threat assessment teams must also have an array of interventions available to them to help develop appropriate action plans based on the level of risk. Depending upon the risk level, an action plan can range from no action needed to a recommendation for the individual to seek professional services, to removal from campus and/or arrest. For example, in cases involving students, team members should be fully aware of campus policies for removing a student from campus, such as interim/summary suspensions and/or expulsion, and who has the authority to invoke these actions. Similarly, any administrators who take action to remove a faculty or staff member should consider policies and laws around leaves and termination. In all cases, including those involving nonaffiliated others, the most appropriate action also may be to ban the individual of concern from campus by issuing a no-trespass order. The team must have steps in place for ongoing monitoring of the individuals to determine if the action plans are effective and if/when such plans may be ceased.

In summary, the threat assessment process must be objective and individualized with careful review of a great deal of information from a variety of sources. Although this is not a complete discussion of all the issues, we hope the information provides readers with some of the critical issues to consider when conducting a threat assessment. To implement and conduct an objective and fact-based threat assessment process, IHEs must have a framework in place, including adequate resources and training. This chapter now turns to the various issues involved in developing a threat assessment team framework.

Campus Threat Assessment Team Framework

As previously mentioned, the process of conducting a threat assessment requires a multidisciplinary team with specific backgrounds,
expertise, and training. A team approach offers the opportunity to
converge information and to "connect the dots" about concerning
behaviors that may be observed by many individuals. In short, teams
enhance communication, ensuring that information can be chan-
neled to one place. Several authors, including Deisinger et al. (2008)
and Dunkle, Silverstein, and Warner (2008), have provided guidance
on developing campus threat assessment teams. Next, we discuss
some of the major issues that campuses may consider in developing and implementing their teams. In particular, we caution against
an inflexible approach to threat assessment. Teams should certainly
have some general structure but enough flexibility to ensure a truly
individualized assessment process tailored to the specific case at
hand. We encourage readers to think of the issues discussed ahead
as general considerations and not an all-inclusive, inflexible model.
In essence, a "one-size-fits-all" assessment process is not recommended and runs counter to a truly individualized approach.

Number/Name of Teams

One of the first components IHEs need to consider is the number of
teams to have. On the one hand, in the interest of efficiency, IHEs
may decide to have one threat assessment team that manages all
persons of concern: students, faculty/staff, and others. On the other
hand, because of some of the different legal and other nuances, campuses may decide to have separate teams for students and for faculty/
staff and nonaffiliated individuals. Although the number of teams
is an essential matter for campuses to consider, given their unique
environments and cultures, it is critical that, no matter how many
teams exist, they communicate among each other. For instance, a
student may be the focus of concern with expressed intent to do
violence toward a faculty member, in which case communication
between separate teams will be important.

An emerging trend on many campuses has been the development
of a spectrum of teams, especially in the case of teams focusing on

students. Specifically, many IHEs conceptualize their teams on a spectrum, from "care teams," which tend to be more focused on providing support to students who do not rise to the level of a threat to the community, to "threat assessment teams," which tend to be more focused on prevention of violence. Although threat assessment may be understood broadly as a process of formally evaluating the degree and nature of a threat in relationship to a specific target, typical college care teams' areas of concern may include psychosocial and behavioral problems that may interfere with adequate and successful functioning but not rise to the level of violence. If unaddressed, these issues might lead to a dangerous outcome for the student or the community.

There are disadvantages to relying exclusively on either a threat assessment team or a care team. Disadvantages of using solely a threat approach may include (a) the team might not find out about cases until there is a serious and acute problem, and (b) given the relative safety of college campuses, the team might actually have little opportunity to meet and may become complacent from lack of practice in doing threat assessment. Care teams, in contrast, may be slow or reluctant to take stronger actions when necessary, such as removing students from school. Care teams also may lack the formal assessment tools to recognize threats or categorize their severity for proper management. In practice, many campuses will choose a hybrid model in which they have multiple teams or identify subsets of a larger team to deal with different sorts of threats.

It is also important that the team name accurately reflect its aim and scope. Gamm, Mardis, and Sullivan (2011) shared findings of a survey of 175 IHEs about campuses' team names across the United States. The most common name was Behavioral Intervention Team (BIT), but other common names included Student Crisis Action Team, Communicating Action Response for Emergency (CARE), Care and Action for Students Team (CAST), Student Protection Response Team (SPRT), Action for Students in Suffering Team (ASIST), Ensuring Action for Students in Emergency (EASE), and Action Crisis Team for Students (ACTS). Most team names had an acronym associated with them, which may be helpful for ease of recognition among campus community members. The most important issue is that the IHE choose a name that reflects the campus team's mission and purpose.

Team Membership, Roles, and Responsibilities

Team membership varies depending upon several factors, including, but not limited to, institutional resources and culture. Typical teams include campus law enforcement, deans of students, student conduct administrators, and/or mental health/counseling. Campus law enforcement or other local police authorities bring their expertise in criminal justice to the table. They also have the ability to access resources at the local, state, and federal levels to gather critical information, including, but not limited to, criminal record history and/or whether the person of concern is a legal firearm owner. In cases involving students of concern, deans of students and/or student conduct administrators offer the ability to access student conduct records to determine if the student has a history of disruptive behavior or other disciplinary issues. They also have expertise in the campus policies around the student disciplinary process to make sure the team does not run counter to campus policies. In the aftermath of the review of the tragedy on the Virginia Tech campus in April 2007, the final report of a review panel on the shootings revealed that there was a great deal of confusion among campus members about what information could or could not be shared (Virginia Tech Review Panel, 2007). Much clarification has been provided to reinforce the fact that a great deal can be shared under the Family Educational Rights and Privacy Act (FERPA), also known as the Buckley Amendment. FERPA is a federal law that protects students' written records, including disciplinary/conduct records, and offers ample leeway for campus administrators to share information on a need-to-know basis and in situations that are a matter of health and safety. As such, deans of students and/or conduct officers are able to share information while remaining within legally sound parameters and should share with other campus officials without hesitation when necessary.

Campus teams also typically have a mental health professional representative, someone from on-campus counseling services or an off-campus consultant. Mental health professionals provide expertise in areas of mental health syndromes, the various laws and standards of care related to the mental health field, and how those issues might come to bear on the threat assessment process. It is critical that the mental health representative on the team not be in a treatment relationship (which may include those supervising treatment providers) with the identified person of concern in order to avoid conflict of interest and dual relationship boundaries. Campus mental health staff are best thought of as sources of expertise rather than information. They may appropriately offer guidance on information provided by other team members, but not reveal information from clinical records protected by state laws and professional ethical guidelines. Campus mental health practitioners may also receive information to help inform treatment or assessment without sharing. It is an important responsibility of all members of the team and especially the team leaders to protect the special confidentiality held by campus mental health services and not push for information. There are several advantages to this approach: (a) Using secondary sources of information supports accuracy; (b) protecting the perception of confidentiality of mental health services encourages students to continue to use counseling services voluntarily, which is paramount for long-term campus health and safety; and (c) making determinations using behavioral data rather than mental health data is likely to be more defensible (and appropriately so) given disability laws. For this reason, it is also important to have a disability law expert on the team.

A campus ADA coordinator or disability services representative is also typically a member of or consultant to threat assessment teams to offer input about laws and practices pertaining to nondiscriminatory actions related to disabilities. Because of special considerations related to visa status, a representative from the campus international office would be able to provide valuable input in cases involving international students of concern. Similarly, because many campuses offer a variety of international opportunities, such as study abroad and research experiences abroad, campus threat assessment teams may consider bringing in representatives from offices overseeing these experiences.

Many campuses have begun hiring case managers within counseling centers and/or student affairs. The main role of case managers is to ensure students do not fall through the cracks, especially when connecting them with off-campus providers. A new professional organization has developed specifically for case managers at colleges and universities, called Higher Education Case Managers Association (HECMA). The development of HECMA points to the growing area of specialization of case managers in postsecondary institutions. Case managers also are becoming more commonplace on threat assessment teams to assist with documentation and other follow-up issues when assessing threat levels of individuals of concern. In fact, the Virginia Tech (Virginia Polytechnic Institute and State University, 2009) Threat Assessment Demonstration Project offers examples of case managers' job descriptions within counseling centers, student affairs, human resources, and teams.

For issues related to faculty and staff who may be of concern on a campus, it is important that teams have representation from human resources. As mentioned earlier, human resources can offer valuable information about employment laws and can access employee files to determine if the individual has a history of troubling behavior. If a campus has an employee assistance program, a representative from that office could be available to offer expertise about and support for employees who are the focus of the team's inquiry. Legal counsel may also be a part of teams or serve as consultants to them. Participation on the team could have disadvantages, however, as information may be privileged and less likely to be shared with the public, in which case the team may defeat its purpose of being able to share information. This is perhaps a subset of a larger danger; for example, team members may become overly deferential to the legalistic perspective with the presence of an attorney. Although such a perspective is valuable, it should be integrated with other threat assessment approaches, and the team should remain conscious of the purpose of both the team and the institution (Lake, 2009).

Finally, other individuals may be asked to join the team as ad hoc members. For example, a chair of an academic department may need to attend and provide information to the team about a faculty member, but the chair would most likely not need to be a permanent member. Also, the team may call upon local, off-campus law enforcement or law enforcement from other areas in cases involving nonaffiliated individuals of concern.

Team Leadership and Training

Somewhat related to the issues of team member roles and responsibilities is the issue of assigning team leadership. Team leaders are responsible for calling the team together and ensuring that the process flows smoothly for determining the level of threat. It is up to each campus to determine who will be the team leader. One option for team leadership would be a campus law enforcement officer, such as the police chief. This would be a wise option for teams that review students, faculty/staff, and nonaffiliated individuals, because campus law enforcement is responsible for the safety of all campus community members. Therefore, the law enforcement officer would have the perspective of the potential threat from all possible angles. For teams specifically focused on students, the dean of students or other similar conduct officer may be a good choice for team leader because of his or her expertise in student conduct. Furthermore, conduct officers are less restricted legally than mental health professionals—for example, when it comes to sharing important information. Some IHEs may decide to have a coleadership format with a campus law enforcement representative and conduct officer.

It would be ill advised to have a mental health professional, such as the counseling center director, as the team leader for a number of reasons. As previously stated, mental health professionals must abide by strict mental health confidentiality laws and, therefore, are extremely limited in the information they can share. Also, putting the counseling center as the lead of a campus threat assessment team runs the risk of perpetuating a myth that all individuals with mental health concerns are dangerous, when a vast majority of them are not. In fact, an individual with mental health issues is more likely to be a victim of a crime than the perpetrator of one (Hiday, Swartz, Swanson, Borum, & Wagner, 1999). Finally, students may become more reluctant to seek out counseling services if they perceive that the counseling center staff oversees the threat assessment team.

Whatever the makeup of a campus team, training and professional development in threat assessment are essential and must be done on an ongoing basis. Campus law enforcement personnel do not necessarily have any training in conducting threat assessment. The same statement could be made regarding conduct officers. Similarly, most mental health professionals in campus counseling services are generalists, with training in assessment concerning suicidality; most, if not all, counseling center mental health professionals do not receive training in conducting threat assessment.

We highly encourage that teams meet even if there are no cases to discuss so as to prevent complacency and to develop group cohesion and trust among the team members. At meetings where no cases are presented, teams could conduct various tabletop exercises, review/debrief case examples, and/or engage in other professional development. Campuses have a wide variety of resources available for training and consultations.

Documentation and Information Sharing

An important part of the planning process in setting up a campus threat assessment team is determining how information will be documented and shared among team members. The information that the team gathers and reviews and the decisions the team makes must be summarized in a record. The individual maintaining the records should have training in documentation practices. In the unlikely event that a case should proceed to a court and/or team records are subpoenaed, an institution will be in a much more legally sound position with high-quality record-keeping practices. In addition, high-quality documentation reflects sound threat assessment practice and decision making.

There are many options for teams regarding documentation, each with pros and cons. An initial question is which party will be the custodian of the records. One option would be for records to be maintained by the dean of students and/or conduct officers. In this case, FERPA would apply to the records and would allow for information to be more easily shared with others on a need-to-know basis. However, this approach would apply only to student cases. An alternative would be to have campus law enforcement be the custodian of the records. In this way, all types of cases could be documented and applicable laws for police records would apply. It is not recommended that campus threat assessment team records be maintained as mental health records for similar reasons mentioned earlier regarding mental health privacy laws.

Teams have a number of options for modes of documentation. One of the guiding principles for the mode of documentation should be ease of information sharing among team members. In addition, whatever mode of documentation is selected, measures must be taken to ensure security and privacy of the information, balanced with the ability to share easily when needed. For these reasons, it is especially unwise to have the counseling center representative or disability offices representative (or others with extra restrictions on information sharing) lead the threat assessment (as discussed earlier) or be responsible for documentation, follow-up, or assessment of the process. Whoever does manage documentation should pay close attention to three critical points of documentation: (a) identification/assessment of risk (the concern and evidence for risk assessment), (b) risk mitigation/prevention (what was done to manage the identified risk), and (c) risk resolution/relocation/alternative action (what was done that led to a state of acceptable risk without further action, and which alternative actions were considered but justifiably rejected). Rigorously including such information is wise from an operational effectiveness perspective and offers the best evidence for having acted rationally and competently in case the legal defensibility of team actions is later questioned (Day Shaw, Mistler, & Nolan, 2014).

Electronic resources are good options for achieving these goals. For example, student conduct cases may be electronically filed, with appropriate access levels, to document other concerns not resulting in sanctions. There are various existing electronic options that campuses can explore, or institutions may choose to develop their own software program for maintaining records. Campuses should note that in many cases information recorded by any means may be considered part of a student's educational record and administrators should have clear policies delineating what does and does not fall into such categories. These categories may later determine a student's right to access his or her information.

Equally, electronic systems, although useful for recording a range of relevant information, are not a panacea; at their best, they accurately record the process of the team, and good recording of a poor process is just that. The mere act of recording information is not a protection. Campus team members are best served by having a clear understanding of procedures and outcomes among members and clear metrics and procedures outlining what sort of information is documented, when it is to be recorded, when an individual warrants a higher level of concern, and what actions are needed in such cases before the situation can be considered resolved. Software or other methods of recording used by the campus team may duplicate or be integrated with judicial software, and yet each component's distinctive purpose must remain clear. It may be appropriate to record some personal information about a student when it is relevant to his or her functioning on campus, such as if the student was reportedly targeting another student based on race, gender expression, or sexual identity, or to clarify appropriate pronouns to be used by team members when communicating with a student (Lennon & Mistler, 2010, 2014). At the same time, resist the temptation to document everything reported to or discussed by the team, such as pseudoassessments of the student's possible mental health concerns by nonprofessionals or undocumented, speculative, or unrelated disability information. Other nonbehavioral or unsubstantial information should be carefully reviewed, lest decisions are perceived to be inappropriately based on (or worse, actually influenced by) such possibly prejudicial grounds.

Beyond the Team: A Public Health/Community Approach

Whatever the team model is, sharing and receiving information between and among the team and IHE stakeholders in a timely manner is a matter of great import. It is critical that campus safety issues not be the sole responsibility of the campus threat assessment team. Certainly, the team plays a critical and central role, but other campus community members play an important role, as well. The whole campus must be involved in implementing an approach to campus safety; risk/threat assessment should also be seen from a public health/community perspective. Campuses can use the example comprehensive framework developed by The JED Foundation (2013). Although The JED Foundation's framework focuses on mental health promotion and suicide prevention, it could be generalized easily to the area of gun violence prevention. It is the entire campus and community's responsibility to create a safety net to identify and report possible threats, support those in need, restrict access to means for violence (see other chapters in this volume for a more thorough discussion), and carry out critical actions at all stages.

One might ask questions such as: Do the campus and broader community know how to recognize a concern? Do they know who to notify? Who notifies those responsible for threat assessment of a concern, and what level does it need to reach to convene the team? What campuswide training/education is needed? Who needs to know how to report? What is the best way to reach out to ensure all campus stakeholders know what to do when they notice unusual behaviors? In a monograph edited by Dunkle (2010), the authors offered a framework and series of chapters describing how to recognize disruptive/

disturbing behavior for campus students, faculty, and staff. In the end, the campus threat assessment team is only as effective as the campus network in which it exists and the support it receives from the community in gathering data and implementing interventions.

Conclusion

There are many factors to consider when developing a campus threat assessment team. Mass shootings have led to a focus on the need for campus teams, and laws mandating their existence have followed in some cases. A broad evolution in the field of risk assessment has helped develop an approach focused on context-dependent threat assessment rather than a singular focus on identifying high-risk individuals. Campus threat assessment and care teams play a critical role and are the center of violence prevention for IHEs. Ultimately, team members, leaders, and campus administrators are faced with the important and difficult task of balancing privacy and disability laws with healthy information sharing and timely interventions based on probabilistic assessment of limited data in response to potential threats. Although names and memberships of campus threat assessment teams vary slightly, there is tremendous agreement, both in the broad structure/membership and in the need for a campus net of stakeholders. The community must be educated about detecting and reporting possible threats to the team. A team must have clear processes and access to a broad base of resources to act on information in a sensible, effective way to reduce the risk of violence on campuses.

References

Americans with Disabilities Act of 1990, Pub. L. No. 101-336, 104 Stat. 328 (1990).

Brunner, J. L., Wallace, D. L., Reymann, L. S., Sellers, J. J., & McCabe, A. G. (in press). College counseling today: Contemporary students and how counseling centers meet their needs. *Journal of College Student Psychotherapy.*

Bryan, C. J., Stone, S. L., & Rudd, M. D. (2011). A practical, evidence-based approach for means restriction counseling with suicidal patients. *Professional Psychology: Research and Practice, 42*(5), 339–346.

Day Shaw, J., Mistler, B. J., & Book, E. (2013, July). *Threat assessment and behavioral intervention teams for higher education.* Workshop at the Annual Convention of the Florida Association of Campus Safety & Security Administrators, Lido Beach, FL.

Day Shaw, J., Mistler, B. J., & Nolan, J. (2014, February). *Care and threat and assessment teams in operation: Preparation in advance of a national mandate.* Workshop at the National Conference on Law and Higher Education, Orlando, FL.

Deisinger, G., Randazzo, M., O'Neill, D., & Savage, J. (2008). *The handbook for campus threat assessment and management teams.* Stoneham, MA: Applied Risk Management.

Drysdale, D., Modzeleski, W., & Simons, A. (2010). *Campus attacks: Targeted violence affecting institutions of higher education.* Washington, DC: U.S. Secret Service, U.S. Department of Homeland Security, Office of Safe and Drug-Free Schools, U.S. Department of Education, and Federal Bureau of Investigation, U.S. Department of Justice. Retrieved from https://www2.ed.gov/admins/lead/safety/campus-attacks.pdf

Dunkle, J. H. (Ed.). (2010). *Dealing with the behavioral and psychological problems of students: A contemporary update.* New Directions for Student Services, no. 128. New York, NY: Wiley.

Dunkle, J. H., Silverstein, Z. B., & Warner, S. L. (2008). Managing violent and other troubling students: The role of threat assessment teams on campus. *Journal of College and University Law, 34*(3), 585–635.

Gamm, C., Mardis, M., & Sullivan, D. (2011, March 29). *Behavioral intervention and threat assessment teams: Exploring reasonable professional responses.* Paper presented at the American College Personnel Association Annual Conference, Baltimore, MD.

Hiday, V. A., Swartz, M. S., Swanson, J. W., Borum, R., & Wagner, H. R. (1999). Criminal victimization of persons with severe mental illness. *Psychiatric Services, 50,* 62–68.

The JED Foundation. (2013). *Balancing safety and support on campus: A guide for campus teams.* New York, NY: Author.

Lake, P. (2009). *Beyond discipline: Managing the modern higher education environment.* Bradenton, FL: Hierophant.

Lennon, E., & Mistler, B. J. (2010). Breaking the binary: Providing effective counseling to transgender students in college and university settings. *Journal of LGBT Issues in Counseling, 4*(1), 228–240.

Lennon, E., & Mistler, B. J. (2014). Cisgenderism. *Transgender Studies Quarterly, 1*(1), 63–64.

Meloy, J. R. (Ed.). (2006). *The scientific pursuit of stalking.* San Diego, CA: Specialized Training Services.

Meloy, J. R., White, S. G., & Hart, S. (2013). Workplace assessment of targeted violence: The development and reliability of the WAVR-21. *Journal of Forensic Sciences, 58*(5), 1353–1358.

Monahan, J., Steadman, H. J., Appelbaum, P. S., Grisso, T., Mulvey, E. P., Roth, L. H., . . . Silver, E. (2006). The classification of violence risk. *Behavioral Sciences & the Law, 24*(6), 721–730.

Section 504 of the Rehabilitation Act of 1973, 34 C.F.R. Part 104. (1973).

OCR Letter to Spring Arbor (December 10, 2010). Retrieved from http://www
.nacua.org/documents/OCRLetter_SpringArborU.pdf

Virginia Polytechnic Institute and State University. (2009, November). *Implementing behavioral threat assessment teams on campus: A Virginia Tech demonstration project*. Blacksburg, VA: Author.

Virginia Tech Review Panel. (2007). *Mass shootings at Virginia Tech: Report of the review panel*. Retrieved from http://cdm16064.contentdm.oclc.org/cdm/ref/collection/p266901coll4/id/904

Vossekuil, B., Fein, R. A., Reddy, M., Borum, R., & Modzeleski, W. (2004, July). *The final report and findings of the safe school initiative: Implications for the prevention of school attacks in the United States*. Retrieved from http://www2.ed.gov/admins/lead/safety/preventingattacksreport.pdf

6 Behavior Intervention and Case Management

Jen Day Shaw and Sarah B. Westfall

ONCE A campus threat assessment/behavior management team assesses a risk or behavior issue, and the team decides that immediate action by law enforcement or others is unnecessary, campuses use a variety of means to address the issue with the individual, to support the community, and to address issues caused by the individual's behavior to create an ongoing safety and support plan that focuses on both the individual and the campus community. The goal of the team is to determine a risk and mitigate that risk before it becomes a crisis. For many campuses, an increasingly challenging aspect of that role is working with and monitoring the behavior of a significant number of students whose behavior is actively or has been a source of concern for the campus.

The student conduct process can be an effective way of addressing significant behavioral problems. It has the benefit of a standard protocol that typically includes procedural or fair process protections and an established threshold for decision making (e.g., preponderance of evidence), is compliant with Americans with Disabilities Act (ADA) issues, and includes an appeal process and experienced decision makers. It also requires that a student be aware of what information is being used by the institution and that the student be able to provide information on his or her behalf. These processes can work especially well if enough time is available and if students are competent to participate in the process. However, in many instances with behavioral issues, the disciplinary process may not be the best choice for the individual or the institution. Peter Lake (2009), in his seminal text *Beyond Discipline: Managing the Modern Higher Education Environment*, wrote, "The best decision-making will occur when an institution of higher education recognizes where, on a continuum, opportunities for resolution of issues lie" (p. 240).

At many institutions of higher education, alternative processes in addition to the student disciplinary process are effectively used in situations involving students of concern. In this chapter, the authors offer insights into some of these nondisciplinary processes and strategies that may be useful. At many colleges the conduct process is one of several ways of addressing troubling student behavior, and it is rarely the only process used.

Behavior intervention typically follows a series of questions or analytical lenses, covered in the previous chapter. A "bottom-line" question for many administrators is whether a student with concerning behavior can safely remain in the campus community. This question focuses on the student's own safety, as well as the safety of others. Secondary questions focus on the level of real or potential disruption the student's presence may cause, reasonable and available resources (student–staff capacity for residential students, general staff time, security/police support, and psychological/counseling center expertise are four prime examples), and the likelihood that the student can progress (behaviorally, personally, and academically) if the student stays in the campus environment. An underlying standard in gauging all of these issues is one of reasonableness: What is reasonable to expect of a student and of an institution in a given set of circumstances?

As mental health issues for college students have become more pronounced in the last 10 years, institutions have developed a range of policies and practices to deal with increasingly complicated student behavior. Policies (e.g., permitting administrative withdrawals) have proliferated, while the benefits of a "case-by-case approach" have simultaneously become more obvious. Though somewhat paradoxical, these approaches reflect the complexity of many student behavioral issues that are emerging on campuses across the country.

Creating a Campus Culture of Care

In the aftermath of the Virginia Tech tragedy, a constant refrain was "no silos of information." Those who examined the situation urged campuses to consider a means of helping faculty, staff, students, and their families report information about students of concern to one location so a threat assessment team can analyze patterns of behavior that might individually be seen as minor. Now fairly prevalent, programs that provide a central point of contact for campuses vary somewhat, but share basic characteristics. An example is the U Matter We Care program at the University of Florida (UF), a public, residential campus of 50,000 students. The U Matter We Care program urges faculty, staff, students, and family members to heed signs of distress and get that person or information about that person to a helping resource. There is one campuswide e-mail address that is monitored 7 days a week. The program was created using a cross-functional, campuswide team which now includes human resources, so employees in distress are funneled through the same contact information. Marketing materials are widely distributed across campus, with a special emphasis on orientations for students, family, and faculty. A student group of ambassadors gives peer presentations on signs of distress and campus resources for student organizations and residence hall floors. The information that comes into the U Matter program is kept in a database that also accesses conduct records, special population records, and threat assessment team records. In this way, as concerns come in through e-mail, by phone, or directly to the office, that information is quickly compared against other issues so the U Matter team or threat assessment team can follow up as appropriate.

The primary message of the program is that being a UF community member means that Gators take responsibility for each other. For this traditional-age population, faculty are most likely to refer students for help; they are followed by referrals from families, who also commonly ask for advice in working with their students. In 2010, 1,611 interactions with U Matter staff took place. During 2012–2013, that number grew to 8,685 interactions, with 3,700 individual students assisted. In 2013–2014, the number of students assisted by the U Matter team increased to 4,335.

Many campuses have instituted similar programs, often with the campus communication regarding a student in distress being directed to a staff member in the dean of students office or to someone in a case manager position. Examples include the University of North Dakota (see und.edu/und-cares), UNCG Cares at the University of North Carolina at Greensboro (see sa.uncg.edu/dean/uncg-cares), and NOVA Cares at the Northern Virginia Community College (see www.nvcc.edu/about-nova/novacares).

The culture of care that is so important to student safety has been a hallmark of smaller institutions since their inception. Given their size and the likelihood that an individual student is known by multiple others at the institution, the culture of care may not be linked to a specified program, but is likely an ingrained aspect of campus culture. For example, DePaul University notes on their dean of students website that "DOS' work can best be conceptualized by four words: recognize, respond, resolve and reassure" (Dean of Students Office, 2015, "About," para. 2). This speaks to the same goals of the broader community campaigns mentioned earlier. Although such a culture may be realized more readily on a small campus than a large one, it is important that small institutions be intentional and plan for an environment of care. Small size is an advantage, but it is not sufficient, especially given the greater resources typically found at a larger institution.

A culture of care includes the expectation that community members will take note of behaviors of concern and get the person in distress or information about that person to a helping resource. This allows the entire campus to take an active role in noticing and taking action regarding students in distress, which gives teams early warning regarding individuals whose behavior can escalate into something that is threatening to self or others. That initial early warning of the potential for harm is crucial in addressing a risk before it causes a crisis.

Determining Risk

When the threat assessment team is analyzing the behavior of a person of concern, there are many ways to gather additional information so the team has a more complete view of past patterns of behavior, indicators of risk, and current state of mind.

A helpful source of information is how the student of concern has interacted throughout campus. This means finding out information such as whether the student lives on or off campus; grades; behavior in class; student organization membership; whether the student has a conduct record; is registered with a disability; or is a member of a specific population, such as veterans, athletes, or international students. Achieving a complete picture of a student's behavior and life increases the effectiveness with which the team can operate as they assess risk.

If the student lives off campus, consider contacting the property manager or landlord. Likewise, valuable information can be gathered from roommates, including behavior in the home; such issues as cleanliness, decorations, and domestic concerns; and how the student interacts with others, which can facilitate the team's ability to effectively analyze behaviors.

Your team may also consider interviewing roommates, friends, a significant other, and/or family. Each campus approaches these conversations according to its unique culture and philosophy. If the threat is significant, the team will have to weigh whether contacting these individuals will exacerbate the situation with the student of concern.

Additional sources of information include student organizations, religious organizations, and employers. The team must constantly balance the need for additional information to create a full picture with the privacy of the individual of concern so as to not paint the student as an object of fear. How the individual interacts with others, whether he or she can maintain healthy relationships, and how capable he or she is of self-management (e.g., succeed at a job and follow through on commitments) are all key pieces of information necessary to threat assessment teams.

Team members may also consider contacting previously attended institutions (e.g., K–12, community college, 4-year university) if applicable. For high schools, having law enforcement/security call the school resource officer can often net valuable information. School administrators in charge of discipline seem to be more likely to speak frankly to a college or university administrator. It can be helpful to remind these sources that under the Family Educational Rights and Privacy Act (FERPA), information can be freely shared regarding a student transferring to an institution.

Social media may also provide a valuable source of information about a student of concern. Postings on a variety of social media platforms can provide a team a sense of what the student is expressing in a given medium, such as whether the postings are "true" thoughts, impulsive inclinations, or a way to "perform" for others who will access the media.

Law enforcement officers are a tremendous help with background checks, although just a criminal history does not give a full picture. Knowing the number and types of interactions with law enforcement can give the team valuable information. Many states have combined systems that allow campus-based officers to see the history of interactions with law enforcement. Awareness of charges filed but never resolved in court can sometimes offer the team helpful information upon which to base their assessment. Major Paul Lester of the police force at the University of North Carolina at Greensboro is a recognized expert in threat assessment. Lester commented,

> Prior contact with law enforcement is a much better indicator for threat assessments than a criminal history. Most law enforcement agencies will not run criminal histories for threat assessments using the National Crime Information Center (NCIC), unless it involves a criminal investigation. The more effective alternative is a data sharing system between law enforcement agencies that can reveal far more information than a criminal history. These systems can provide information about every collective contact a person has with law enforcement. The data sharing systems are usually regional and capable of spanning multiple jurisdictions with a single search. Some examples include ONESolution Public Safety and Justice Software (formerly OSSI's Police 2 Police [P2P]), Southern Software's Rambler, and Tritech's Inform. These systems are ideal for threat assessments because they can help to establish a pattern of behavior based on contact with law enforcement. (personal communication, July 14, 2014)

If your campus does not have law enforcement, consider creating a memorandum of understanding (MOU) with local law enforcement. An MOU between an institution and local law enforcement is an agreement regarding issues such as jurisdiction, the interplay between the conduct system and the court system, access to campus buildings, notification to both parties, and much more. As an example of an MOU, the state of New Jersey provides a model for its institutions (New Jersey Department of Law & Public Safety and the New Jersey Department of Education, 2011). In addition to memoranda, some campuses include local law enforcement on their threat assessment teams to more closely connect the two resources.

As the team gathers information, there is a constantly evolving process of evaluating the information and its source, what that information means for the overall assessment of risk, and how that information impacts the plan the team develops. For example, finding out a student is currently hospitalized involuntarily will give the team some time to determine a plan. However, if the team learns that the student's behavior is escalating and is negatively impacting others, alternative options will likely be chosen.

Finally, discretion is an important part of determining risk. Compared with many other segments of society, college students have unusual patterns of behavior when it comes to their schedules, the fluidity of their personal relationships, their use of alcohol and other drugs, their access to social media, and their intense exposure to a constantly changing environment (new people, new ways of thinking and seeing). The assessment of risk must be done with full knowledge of the unique context of college in general and of specific campuses in individual cases.

Nondisciplinary Strategies

For students identified as at-risk or a potential threat to themselves or the community, a range of options is available. We outline a few here, in ascending order of intensity, as a way of illustrating the flexibility institutions have (and, perhaps, can create) in responding to complex student behavior.

As options are considered, some primary questions will guide administrative thinking and decision making: Is there an imminent threat? (If yes, then law enforcement is called immediately.) What resources do we have to mitigate risk and help the individual? Who else is impacted by the individual's behavior and how can we support them?

Students can emerge as at-risk or as potential threats for many reasons, and it is imperative that each situation be treated as unique. For example, if a student has emerged as at-risk due to poorly managed mental illness, the approach will likely be quite different from a student who has been identified due to ongoing substance abuse issues. A student with a significant eating disorder requires a different approach than a student who has engaged in stalking behavior.

There may also be relevant policies that address specific behaviors. Most campuses have policies that define and limit weapons on campus, for example. There may not be relevant policies in play for students who are noncompliant with medication regimens (a source of behavioral difficulty for some). If such policies are present, they need to be a factor in administrative decision making.

Finally, the context of the institution is important. A traditional-aged residential student may manifest problematic issues differently than a veteran, a commuting student, or a distance learner. As the team gathers information about the person of concern and derives plans, it is important to take into account those contextual variables that might make actions or the likelihood of violence a greater concern. In addition, the institution will have different norms and values as well as resources. Knowing your own campus and its norms around issues such as involvement of legal counsel, the threshold at which a Clery warning is sent out, notification of external law enforcement, and so on will help the team as decisions are made in quickly evolving situations.

Early Response

Direct, concrete conversation about problematic behavior is an appropriate response in a variety of situations that do not entail violence. This may particularly be helpful to students who perceive social cueing in a nontypical way (e.g., students on the autism spectrum) or who are new to an American college environment. Such discussions review the behavior in question, describe why it is problematic in the perception of others, and include concrete strategies for avoiding it in the future (e.g., imposing self-limits on "air time" during class discussion, addressing faculty members in a particular way, bathing regularly, standing a given distance from others, lowering the volume of one's voice). In part, this is a process of helping a student acclimate to an unfamiliar academic and social culture.

Student affairs administrators sometimes receive calls from faculty members with concerns about difficult classroom behavior, ranging from unconventional or abrupt comments to disruption to hostility. Coaching faculty members on how to have direct, concrete discussions with students may be helpful, with additional help offered if the faculty–student conversation does not result in changed behavior.

There may be gender-related issues at play in some cases. If so, the direct, concrete conversation may be most effectively conducted by a person who is of the same gender as the student, or conducted as a "tag team" that includes a person of the student's gender. As an example, having a male student talk with a male staff member about the student's interactions or perceived pattern of behavior with women can be extraordinarily effective.

One of the major benefits of this approach is that as a result of engaging the student in considering his or her behavior, the staff member can further assess key factors, such as self-awareness, responsibility taking, defensiveness, and the ability to make a change in behavior, which may be all that is needed. From a developmental perspective, the task is to focus on perceptions and consequences that stretch beyond the immediate needs or intentions of the student in question. Larger goals may include building empathy and raising awareness. In short, direct conversations are both a response and an additional opportunity for assessment. Documentation of the discussion, information about next steps if problematic behavior persists, and planned follow-up by staff are all important to the success of early responses.

Consultation

Complicating issues, such as mental illness, substance abuse/addiction, trauma recovery, and neurodiversity, may be confirmed or surface during assessment. In such cases, direct, concrete discussion of the complicating factors, including the student's plans/resources combined with the institution's ability to provide reasonable support, must be assessed. Such discussions may include receiving the student's permission to consult with healthcare or mental health providers, on or off campus. They may also involve contact with parents or family members. This contact is ideally conducted with permission from the student but may be done without if there is a significant and/or immediate health or safety concern. A question at the core of such a discussion is whether there are or can be reasonable efforts to effectively correct or mitigate the behavior.

As an example, a student who has disclosed a mental illness, shared the information that she is no longer engaged in treatment for it, and has developed a pattern of problematic behavior is a good candidate for consultation. If the problematic behavior involves placing unreasonable demands on friends in a manipulative way, that may be a good time to talk with the student in a direct, concrete way about the information available and to seek permission to consult with the student's care providers or family. If the behavior is severe or pervasive and raises concerns about the student's health and safety, a team member may contact a family member without permission.

Ongoing communication and information sharing, along with a system of monitoring (e.g., scheduled "check-in" visits with a staff member), are required to make a consultative strategy work. Defining clear benchmarks or expectations may also be helpful. It is important to document the discussion, information about next steps if problematic behavior persists, and planned follow-up by staff.

Faith-based institutions may have additional, consultative remedies rooted in denominational or institutional doctrine or in cultural expectations. The same may also be true of tribal colleges and other institutions with strong cultural identities, norms, and supports.

Leave of Absence

Time away from the institution is often a helpful nondisciplinary strategy for dealing with problematic behaviors. Leaves can range from a short period of time (a few days to a week) to multiple academic terms. Ideally, a student will choose a leave on his or her own, often with the support of family or mental health providers. It is also important that each institution understand and define its own ability to institute a mandatory leave of absence when necessary if a student does not opt to withdraw willingly. Though leaves vary widely, there are some things they have in common: They involve a complete separation of the student from the institution for a given period of time, they may include conditions to be met for reinstatement (typically for longer-term leaves), and they are nondisciplinary in nature. They may also entail formalized communication between the institution and the student's care providers.

The benefit of a leave, especially if the student opts for one, is that it provides a true "time-out" that may help a student step back from the issues that are problematic and get some perspective and some substantive help. Making the hard decision to leave is something a struggling student can feel good about in the midst of a difficult time period. A leave can also provide some relief to friends, roommates, and staff who are affected by the student's behavior.

Law Enforcement

Contacting campus or local law enforcement is not, by definition, a student disciplinary matter for all institutions. Disciplinary or not, when a threshold related to the safety of a student or others in the community is reached, law enforcement should be contacted. On many, but not all, campuses, legal proceedings occur in parallel with campus discipline. Should nondisciplinary responses prove ineffective or be unwarranted in an individual case, teams are advised to consider using the campus discipline process, including provisions for interim suspensions and administrative withdrawals. Occasionally, such consideration may entail consultation with legal counsel. The essential consideration in using the discipline process is whether the behavior in question is addressed by the student code of conduct or other existing policies. However, in many cases, the disciplinary process can take some time. Teams will need to weigh this factor as they consider options. In addition, teams often struggle with using the campus code of conduct when they know that the behavior is likely a result of untreated mental illness. Having someone who is ill go through the conduct process that potentially results in a permanent conduct record is not always palatable, although the behavior must be addressed in some way.

Case Management

Case managers are used in various fields including those related to social work, health care, and other helping professions (e.g., the Case Management Society of America at www.cmsa.org). This social work framework and approach is directly applicable to higher education. Similar work has been done quite routinely by student affairs professionals who seek to help students and their families identify and prioritize the issues and the resources that can assist in their time of need. The utility of a case management approach is increasingly evident in higher education. Regardless of whether designated case managers or existing staff are fulfilling the functions, the approach can be very helpful.

Case manager, care team member, and assistant dean are three of the many titles used to denote the individual who serves as the primary coordinator of follow-up and monitoring for the campus behavior intervention team or student life entity. At small colleges, this role is not usually defined separately from the overall position description. Typically, the staff member uses a "social work whole person" approach so issues related to academics, personal relationships, living arrangements, finances, goal setting, use of resources, and more are addressed as part of the fundamental goal of student success. Many case managers regularly check in with students of high concern so changes in patterns of behavior are immediately noted and brought to the team's attention for analysis.

Case managers work to develop reasonable and effective success plans for students of concern. They will often consult with colleagues with relevant expertise (e.g., counseling, residential life, student health) in order to develop a plan. Though plans vary due to circumstances and resources, they share a focus on actions that will help a student successfully remain enrolled and, ideally, progress at the institution. Plans typically include requirements for the student (with the assistance of a case manager) to identify needs, use available resources, develop skills and build capacity, facilitate communication between care providers and the institution, and establish personal contingency or crisis protocols. Plans may also include an evaluative component in which progress is noted and verified by care providers or through self-reporting/reflection by the student. Some plans may be very specific. For example, a plan might require that a student connect weekly with the campus counseling center, that the student meet twice a week with the case manager, that the student meet every 2 weeks with each faculty member to fully understand academic progress, and that documentation of a required appointment with the health center be received by a specified authority. Monitoring of plan adherence and progress usually rests with the case manager. As with the plan itself, monitoring can vary greatly, from daily to monthly reviews, with or without communication beyond the student, and with or without initiation by the student.

The success of a plan can be assessed in a variety of ways. Compliance with the plan, academic performance, improved social relations, and better health are examples of success indicators. In the longer term, students' ability to stay enrolled and out of the student disciplinary process might be important indicators of success.

Such information may also be valuable should a student's behavior escalate and ultimately need to be addressed through the student conduct process.

Case managers work closely with on- and off-campus resources and commonly make referrals to counseling services and other units. For example, students with interpersonal communication limitations might be referred to the office of student activities/involvement or the community service office in an effort to create an unintimidating way in which to engage with others. Many case managers develop success plans with students. The plans are based on identifying the issues facing the student, helping the student prioritize those issues, and then determining resources and action steps to address each issue. Students who are in severe distress will likely receive a more directive plan, whereas those who are capable will be supported in learning how to advocate for themselves and reach their own goals.

The choice of who will act as case manager varies greatly depending upon the institution. At smaller institutions, the chief student affairs officer may play this role. At larger institutions, one or more staff may have the case manager function as the sole role. Case managers can be housed in different units, including residential life, the dean of students' office, and the counseling center. It should be noted that a case manager who is part of the counseling center serves a different role from that being described here. In addition to student success, the most important role of a case manager is communicating to the threat assessment team the current status of the student of concern and any warning signs (e.g., communication from family or faculty) that have arisen. This allows the team to act swiftly in determining if a threat to the student or the broader community is imminent. Due to the greater confidentiality restrictions in a counseling center, a case manager housed there cannot serve in this vital role.

Many case managers have a traditional student affairs background and focus their efforts on making connections throughout campus in order to best help students of concern succeed. Such relationships include financial aid (e.g., emergency aid programs, appealing the loss of financial aid due to a lack of forward progress), academic department heads (e.g., student attendance in classes, waivers of problematic courses/assignments, modification of requirements), disability services, housing and residential life (e.g., modifications to living arrangements, having hall staff check in more frequently), religious life, advising, and others.

Competencies for a case manager include the following:

> ➤ The ability to build strong, collegial relationships across campus in order to devise a successful plan and monitor behavior and compliance with the plan (including the ability to navigate between the various cultures on a campus—e.g., law enforcement, faculty, counseling)
> ➤ The ability to build rapport with students and families
> ➤ The ability to quickly and creatively identify options and implement a complex plan with multiple moving parts
> ➤ The ability to communicate clearly and concisely
> ➤ The ability to understand higher education, including the policies and laws associated with case management and threat assessment

The case manager model offers expertise, dedicated focus, and centralized response and resources for students, institutions, and families who are in difficult circumstances. Good case management includes a wide array of tools, including many nondisciplinary processes as well as formal disciplinary and crisis protocols. As student behavior becomes more complex, case managers with expertise and devoted time will become more valuable to colleges and universities and to students.

Working With Family Members

The cooperation and support of family members exists on a continuum, from incredibly helpful to actively working against the goals of the institution. Campus culture varies greatly in regard to whether families are engaged in the threat management process. It is advisable for teams to talk through the prudence of involving family members, with the default option being working with family members. Often, family members are able to provide information that is significant and relevant to the determination of threat, including past medical history, current state of mind, habits, family resources, family influence on decision making, known acquaintances, substance abuse, and more. Teams should carefully select who will establish a relationship with family members as a way to receive ongoing information. Helping families understand the institution's concern for their student, as well as the campus community, is a wise approach.

In addition, helping them understand that the institution's goal is to help their student be successful can help influence their willingness to share information. Particularly if a student is involuntarily hospitalized, having the family engaged with the institution can provide valuable information about medication, state of mind, release date, and plan upon release.

For students who are being monitored, family can be helpful in noticing behavior changes, spending patterns, lack of follow-through with care, and other warning signs that the student may be moving toward a more negative state.

Working With Faculty

The team should think carefully about how and when to involve faculty. Faculty members will react in a variety of ways to news that a student is of concern or to a request for ongoing information. Selecting a team member to consistently interact with faculty and to adeptly explain the role of the team in keeping the student and community safe is an important choice. Providing clarity to faculty partners about what information can be shared, about their desired role, and about support that they may seek is essential.

Faculty members may provide substantive information about academic performance, behavior in the classroom, changes in behavior over time, and career goals. Insightful faculty can often provide information regarding interactions with authority figures, interactions with peers, examples of writing, comments and demeanor in class, hygiene, and attendance. If they have a personal connection to the student, they may also provide helpful contextual information gleaned from conversations with the student over time. The point person should also be aware of which faculty will want periodic updates, what should be shared, and what should remain private.

Strategizing Success Plans and Monitoring

A point person or case manager should be responsible for meeting with the student of concern, identifying issues that require attention, prioritizing and matching those issues with appropriate resources, and setting up a plan with a time line to monitor progression. Having a savvy, sensitive individual periodically seeing a student of concern; checking with alternative sources of information, like family and faculty; and documenting compliance with a care plan is essential. If this person is not a member of the behavioral intervention team, giving regular updates to the team chair is important to ensure consistency in follow-up. A clear process for the point person to learn team concerns and plans should also be in place.

Because students vary widely, as do their concerns and problems, plans for supporting them can be creative in approach, strategy, and use of campus and community resources. The point person for case management, in consultation with other campus resource people, should be guided by two questions: What will enable this student to succeed here? Can risk/negative impact to the community be mitigated and addressed? Though there are obvious resources and strategies (e.g., counseling support, healthcare compliance, academic coaching) that will help many students, there are many options open to creative professionals in supporting the student in distress. These may involve athletics and recreation colleagues, student organizations and activities, civic engagement, connections to specific peer resources, or involvement in the community beyond the campus. They will likely involve a variety of strategies for communication and documentation as well, including in-person contact, electronic "check-ins," student self-assessment, and a regimen of documentation by campus and community partners. The key is to focus on what will help a student succeed, and to employ a range of tools in that process. Each plan should be individualized, monitored, and documented.

Case Studies

Teams may find it helpful to use scenarios like those in this chapter in order to assess protocol, the ability to secure necessary information, resources, communication patterns, and team dynamics. Each of the scenarios is a real-life example provided by institutions. The authors suggest going through each case study as if it were an actual case as a tabletop exercise. Have each team member relate what his or her role would be in such a scenario, sources of information, documentation, and possible options for next steps. If possible, have someone from another institution who is trained in threat assessment observe the tabletop and provide feedback.

1. Johnny is chronically suicidal. He has been hospitalized multiple times for attempts, although none have happened on campus. Each previous attempt has been by overdosing on medication. He is a highly successful student, with a 3.9 GPA in chemistry. He lives on campus by himself. His family is influential. The team has just been alerted by Johnny's mother, an attorney, that he has been hospitalized again.

2. A custodial worker reports to campus safety that Martin has some weird drawings in his trash, including what looks like cartoons of Martin shooting students in the student union. Words like "Plan Nitro" and "Them Before Me" are written on the paper.

3. A faculty member reports to the dean that Brittany has become slovenly, distrustful, and antisocial. She has several new tattoos and has written several dark essays, including one in which she talks of "taking out" the bullies who have been "tormenting" her.

4. Phoenix is a popular student who suddenly begins describing himself as a god of war with the power to heal. He regularly stands on a table in the cafeteria to do so. Other students aren't sure what to think. He attends class, obeys the rules, and refuses to visit the counseling center.

5. Rex has made threats to two men on his floor. He is not well known to campus, having just transferred from a school out of state. His roommate has requested a room move. Faculty describe him as "creepy" and "intense."

6. Betty is constantly at the rec center. Although 5 feet, 9 inches tall, she looks about 90 pounds. Today, she passed out when working out. She reported to staff that she had not eaten that day. It was 2:00 p.m. and she had been working out since 12:30 p.m.

7. Leslie reports that her former boyfriend Will refuses to accept their breakup. She shares that he constantly texts her, shows up at her classes, and has been leaving her weird gifts. The person she went out with this weekend had his car keyed and a pocketknife was found in his flat tire.

Conclusion

Behavior intervention and case management are taking more and more time on campuses across the country. The work is complex and can involve rapidly changing circumstances, incomplete information, serious and/or persistent behavioral problems that affect individual students and the larger community, and limited resources. The benefits of competent behavior intervention and case management range from retaining students who might have otherwise left the institution to protecting the campus community from a person intending to do harm. Competent work can also lead to developing a campus culture that is supportive of students who are struggling and that instills confidence in the broader community.

In developing or improving effective behavior intervention and case management processes, a variety of resources and practices may be helpful. Assessment is an obvious initial step. What are examples of institutional "misses" and successes with behavioral issues, and what can be learned from them? Are there patterns to what works well and what doesn't? Is the right expertise available to the point person or team responding to concerning behavior? Is there a process that is well understood by the people responsible for ensuring that it is employed?

Sister institutions can provide valuable models, experience, and training. Because context is so important, looking to similar institutions for ideas and protocols can be helpful. Exchanging training and expertise, enabling colleagues in similar positions to share experiences, and sharing brainpower to address common problems can be fruitful. An extended lunch meeting with area colleagues, for example, can facilitate a great deal of sharing and strategizing. Similarly, attending conferences and conference sessions that focus on issues related to behavior intervention is a way to hone expertise and broaden the repertoire of options available to case managers. As with many emerging issues, staying up to date with federal regulations and professional/scholarly writing on related matters is another way of improving the work in this area.

Consulting with off-campus resources and expertise can also strengthen institutional processes. Local resources related to mental health, law enforcement, and physical and spiritual health, for example, can ensure that campus processes are comprehensive and inclusive while providing some creative options for the case manager. Governmental agencies, including the Federal Bureau of Investigation and Secret Service, can provide specialized training to campus teams.

In general, seek to continually improve your services, protocol, relationships, and resources. Focus time, energy, and resources on these valuable and necessary tasks. Be assured that the work you do is valuable and vital to your campus community's well-being.

More specific recommendations include the following:

1. Create a behavioral intervention team that trains together, including tabletop exercises. Establish methods of operating, communicating, documenting the process, and assessing students of concern.
2. Create a campaign that encourages campus community members to share information with a designated point of contact.
3. Provide campus training on signs of distress and helping resources.
4. Establish a database of information accessible to a member(s) of the team that tracks pieces of information about students of concern to ensure that silos of information do not exist.
5. Establish relationships with potential sources of referral, information, and resources that can actively support students of concern.
6. Consider memoranda of understanding with area law enforcement and mental health hospitals.
7. Know your state laws regarding involuntary hospitalization and remain current with the Office for Civil Rights "Dear Colleague" letters, and legal parameters for the work you do.
8. Determine protocols for the team that include whether they recommend or decide, authority to act, and purview.
9. Ensure that the appropriate institutional leaders understand the processes for behavioral intervention and that they are informed when they need to be.

Select campus examples of marketing campaigns and case management are shown in Table 6.1.

Table 6.1 Select Campus Examples of Marketing Campaigns and Case Management

University	Population	Case manager? Which office?	How many case managers?	Marketing campaign?
Auburn University	20,200	Yes, student conduct office	1	None
Duke University	15,400	Yes, dean of students office	3	DukeReach: studentaffairs.duke.edu/dos/dukereach
Texas A&M University	58,800	Yes, dean of student life office	2	Tell Somebody Campaign: tellsomebody.tamu.edu
University of Alabama	34,900	Yes, dean of students office	2	New campaign being developed
University of Florida	50,000	Yes, dean of students office	4	U Matter We Care: umatter.ufl.edu
University of Kentucky	28,928	Yes, dean of students office	2	Community of Concern: uky.edu/concern
University of Virginia	21,000	Yes, counseling and psychological services; also associate/assistant deans from dean of students office		Just Report It portal: Virginia.edu/safercommunity

References

Lake, P. (2009). *Beyond discipline: Managing the modern higher education environment.* Bradenton, FL: Hierophant.

New Jersey Department of Law & Public Safety and the New Jersey Department of Education (2011). *A uniform state memorandum of agreement between education and law enforcement officials.* (2011). Retrieved from http://www.state.nj.us/education/schools/security/regs/agree.pdf

7 Timely Warning and Crisis Communication

Jeanna Mastrodicasa and Greg Nayor

At THE time of the first mass shooting on a college campus in 1966 at the University of Texas at Austin, the best method for mass communication was the hope that a radio station would broadcast a warning informing students to stay off campus (Todd, 2013). Today, there are several mandates that require timely warnings and multiple avenues of planned communication that meld technology and traditional means, such as locked doors, police reports, or a bullhorn, to help keep a campus community informed and safe (Todd, 2013).

As the role of technology within a college student's life has become increasingly prevalent, there have been necessary shifts in the processes, frequency, and expectations of communication. The pace of change related to technology and its use is quite fast, and preferences change quickly. For example, a study in 2006 by Junco and Mastrodicasa (2007) showed that the median number of times college students talk on the phone to their parents was 1.5 per day, a drastic change in communication frequency compared to previous generations. Today, technology has provided numerous avenues to communicate with college students, and their preferences are evolving as quickly as the devices.

Technological Devices

Most undergraduate college students come to campus with multiple technology devices—usually between two and four—for personal and academic use (Dahlstrom, Walker, & Dziuban, 2013). Ownership of smartphones and tablets increased the most among all devices between 2012 and 2013 for undergraduate students, and ownership of these devices exceeds that of the general adult population (Dahl-strom et al., 2013; Pew Research Center, 2014). The American adult population is certainly mobile friendly: 90% of Americans own a cell phone, 58% own a smartphone, and 42% own a tablet (Pew Research Center, 2014). One study estimates smartphone usage among U.S. college students at 89% (Negrea, 2014).

Despite the popularity of these technological devices, studies show there are still ownership and proficiency differences within the college student population. Junco, Merson, and Salter (2010) found a digital divide of differences among gender, race, and income with college students' use of technology. For example, one difference was that female White students owned cell phones at a rate more than twice that of male African American students (Junco et al., 2010). Also, Junco et al. (2010) found that race, sex, and income also proved to have differential impacts. They determined that being female, being African American, and/or being from the highest income brackets were positively predictive of the number of text messages sent and the amount of time spent talking on a cell phone per week. In a different study, Dahlstrom et al. (2013) reported that students who are male or White tend to have more Internet devices than those who are female or non-White. Accordingly, college administrators need to remain sensitive that college students do not all possess the same connection to technology and vary within their population.

E-mail remains a prevalent form of communication with college students as a formal channel with an archiving system that is both reliable and secure (Kolowich, 2011). Institutions of higher education historically developed their own e-mail systems but have explored using outside providers and cloud services to support e-mail services for students (Kolowich, 2011, 2012). However, the use of e-mail as a means to communicate with college students has been questioned in the past few years as an unreliable method because students may not check their e-mail regularly, if at all (Rubin, 2013). A study by Junco found that students use e-mail only 6 minutes per day, compared to 31 minutes on social networking (Rubin, 2013). Some institutions have announced that they consider e-mail official notification, and professors have mandated that students check e-mail daily by placing this requirement in syllabi (Rubin, 2013).

Texting is another popular means of communication, with 81% of American adults using their phones to text, as compared to 52%

using them to e-mail in 2013 (Duggan & Smith, 2014). Even during class, 90% of students in a study reported using their phones for non-class activities (Jaschik, 2013; McCoy, 2013). McCoy (2013) also found that undergraduates reported using their devices for nonclass purposes 11 times a day on average, compared to graduate students, who used them 4 times a day (Jaschik, 2013).

In fact, people's connections to their cell phones has grown quite intense over the past few years, along with their major adoption of use. Pew Research Center (2014) reported that 44% of cell owners have slept with their phone next to their bed because they wanted to make sure they didn't miss any calls, text messages, or other updates during the night. Even when they do not notice their phone ringing or vibrating, 67% of cell owners find themselves checking their phone for messages, alerts, or calls (Pew Research Center, 2014).

Social Media

The term *social media* encompasses websites that allow users to connect to one another based on shared interests, activities, or characteristics. Users can post their personal information and pictures on a profile page, which displays a list of the user's connections (Junco & Cole-Avent, 2008; Junco & Mastrodicasa, 2007). These sites provide various forms of communication between users, such as wall posts, comments, pictures, and private messages, as well as methods to tag photos in order to identify those in the picture (Junco & Cole-Avent, 2008; Junco & Mastrodicasa, 2007).

Beyond the social networking sites themselves, the popularity of mobile technology with cell phones impacts college students in other ways. Having near-constant mobile access provides access to the Internet from any location; anonymous communication; instant information sharing; and quick, easy photograph taking and sharing (Mastrodicasa & Metellus, 2013). Students are not only using social media sites at home on a computer but also accessing these sites via their cell phones (Mastrodicasa & Metellus, 2013).

Facebook is the most popular social media site overall, with 802 million daily users as of March 2014; 609 million of those daily active users are connecting to Facebook with a mobile device (Facebook, 2014). Twitter is also popular, with 255 million monthly active users and 78% of Twitter active users on mobile devices (Twitter, 2014). As of 2013, 84% of individuals aged 19–29 used Facebook, compared to the 31% who used the social media site Twitter (Duggan & Smith, 2013). Junco's 2013 study of college students found that students used the site with equal frequency, regardless of their backgrounds, spending an average of 101 minutes a day on Facebook. However, he found differences in how students use Facebook; for example, women were more likely to use Facebook for communication, African Americans were less likely to use Facebook to check up on their friends, and students from lower socioeconomic levels were less likely to use Facebook for communication and sharing (Junco, 2013). Accordingly, social media are important communication channels for college students, but their impact and preferred use varies across student subpopulations.

Crisis Communication

A college campus community is made up of students, faculty, and staff, with key stakeholders that include parents and students' families, the local community, law enforcement, and many others; thus, effectively and efficiently communicating about a crisis on campus is a challenge (Lawson, 2007; Rollo & Zdziarski, 2007; Zdziarski et al., 2007). Generally speaking, the speed of disseminating critical information to various constituencies is a significant factor in evaluating the success of crisis communication (Lawson, 2007; Rollo & Zdziarski, 2007). For example, administrators should anticipate landlines becoming nonfunctional in storms, but mobile networks often stay up. Thus, social networking and mobile applications can be used to keep the lines of communication open for emergency crews, first responders, and citizens (West & Valentini, 2013). The importance of including communications in planning and operations of a campus crisis cannot be overstated (Haddow & Haddow, 2014; Lawson, 2007; Rollo & Zdziarski, 2007; Zdziarski et al., 2007).

As Harper, Paterson, and Zdziarksi (2006) aptly noted, one of the most fundamental pieces of the crisis management process is ensuring that communications are timely, consistent, and accurate. Although this may seem obvious today to higher education administrators, that was not the case less than a decade ago. Prior to 2003, colleges and universities, as well as many other agencies, were using different methods for managing a crisis. It was not until 2003 that then-president Bush issued Homeland Security Presidential Directive-5 (HSPD-5) mandating that the Department of Homeland Security develop the National Incident Management System to ensure that all government, nongovernment, and private sector entities could coordinate responses during a crisis (HSPD-5, 2003). The resulting incident command system, a necessary implementation for a successful crisis management team (CMT), outlines specific roles for each potential crisis, led by an incident commander. Perhaps the most important of these roles is that of the public information officer (PIO), who is responsible for disseminating timely, consistent communication, both during and after the crisis.

Another important component, a piece of federal legislation, is the Jeanne Clery Disclosure of Campus Security Policy and Campus Crime Statistics Act (Clery Act), which requires all colleges and universities that participate in federal financial aid programs to maintain and disclose information about crime on and near their respective campuses (Clery Center, 2014). Named for a 19-year-old Lehigh University freshman who was raped and murdered in her campus residence hall in 1986, the law was created in response to the outrage over unreported crimes on college campuses (Clery Center, 2014). In addition to keeping a log and reporting annual crime statistics for a specific list of serious crimes, the Clery Act requires campuses to issue "timely warnings" about Clery Act crimes that pose a serious or ongoing threat to students and employees, in a manner likely to reach all members of the campus community (Clery Center, 2014).

Beyond the timely warnings mandate, the Clery Act also requires institutions to use an "emergency response" to the campus community about a "significant emergency or dangerous situation involving an immediate threat to the health or safety of students or employees occurring on the campus" (Clery Center, 2014). An emergency response expands the definition of *timely warning* as it includes both Clery Act crimes and other types of emergencies (e.g., a fire or infectious disease outbreak) (Clery Center, 2014).

During a crisis, or a suspected incident, the 2008 revisions to the Clery Act are very clear about the requirements of the institution by distinguishing between a timely warning and an emergency notification. The former remains relatively unchanged and is triggered by a "Clery-reportable act" that has occurred on campus, on immediately accessible adjacent property, or on noncampus property, such as a Greek house, that is shared with a previously identified campus crime officer, such as someone from campus safety, the dean of students, and even resident assistants. The latter, however, is much broader and addresses any potential threat to the health and well-being of the campus community, regardless of the nature of the emergency and/or location. A simple example of an incident that would qualify as an emergency notification, but not a timely warning, would be a severe weather alert (Carter, n.d.). It is, therefore, imperative that a CMT provides standards for managing both timely warnings and emergency notifications during an incident.

The 2007 shooting of 32 victims at Virginia Tech led to allegations that the university failed to provide a timely warning to the campus, as mandated by the Clery Act. This incident led to a new understanding of the term *timely notification*. In general, it is expected, both legally and ethically, that as soon as the institution has any indication of any potential threat to the campus community, the threat and directions for ensuring personal safety must be adequately communicated to the campus in a clear, direct, and succinct manner. Although this task seems straightforward, there remain many unanswered questions about these criteria, such as: (a) Who is responsible for these communications? (b) What information, while the incident develops, should be shared? and (c) How does the institution ensure that as many members of the campus community as possible are notified?

Perhaps a common misconception is that the PIO is necessary only during a crisis situation and its aftermath. At that point, however, whatever information is shared comes too late. Effective communication means preparing the institution of higher education for how the campus community and local authorities will respond during an incident and what is expected by them. It is unreasonable to believe that community members unaccustomed to dealing with a traumatic situation will recall emergency procedures during a crisis event. To that end, it is critical that succinct information is made available in a variety of formats at all times. Students should carry ID cards with them that list critical information on the back, such as emergency contacts, shelter-in-place instructions, or other basic information; this may serve as a quick, potentially lifesaving reminder. Additionally, whereas posting the actual response procedures by the CMT may be counterproductive, displaying posters that quickly remind people to "Run, Hide, or Fight," as well as what number to call, may prove effective. Many colleges and universities continue to develop smartphone and tablet apps for ensuring community members stay informed.

Although it may seem rather obvious, the most effective way to ensure the campus community receives vital information is to create simple, straightforward templates that may be quickly updated to include time, date, and specifics, and keeping the templates in an easily accessible location. These templates apply to not only electronically sent written messages but also audio announcements that may be delivered on a public address (PA) or paging system. Additionally, there should be printed templates of notifications hung in various locations in the event the server breaks down or there is a loss of electrical power. Several years ago, a fairly significant earthquake occurred in the Washington, D.C., area and was felt all along the East Coast. As East Coast institutions were not prepared for such an incident, both land and cell phone lines clogged and servers jammed. A natural disaster is not reportable as part of a Clery statistic, but it may affect as many, if not more, members of the community than an active shooter. Preparing for an emergency means having simple, straightforward templates available for both high- and low-tech avenues of communication.

Haddow and Haddow (2014) recommended principles of a successful communications strategy through all four phases of emergency management—"mitigation, preparedness, response, and recovery" (p. 71). Those principles include the following:

1. Focus on the needs of the customers.
2. Make a commitment to effective communications.
3. Make communications an integral part of planning and operations.
4. Be transparent in your communications.
5. Ensure your information is accurate.
6. Release information in a timely manner.

7. Make yourself, your staff, and technical experts where appropriate available and accessible.
8. Create an emotional connection with your audience.
9. Build a partnership with the media and the public using social media. (p. 71)

When applying these principles to incidents such as a campus shooting, the importance of instant, accurate, and multipronged communication strategies is clearly evident.

Building Redundancy

Assuming that all services are functional, a campus should possess several channels of communication during a crisis. There is, and should be, a certain level of redundancy built into these systems to ensure that as many people receive critical information as possible. Relying on only one system, such as e-mail or text alert, could prove problematic during a crisis. On the most basic level, the campus should invest in, and have at its disposal, the following communication mediums:

- E-mail
- Text alert
- Web/portal announcements
- Social media (Facebook, Twitter, etc.)
- Siren/PA system

The siren/PA system may be the most cost prohibitive, but it may also be the most valuable. In a scenario in which an active shooting is occurring in a high-rise building of an urban campus, for example, the most efficient manner to warn community members to shelter in place will be through a PA system and/or siren.

As technology use has increased, so has the ability to deliver services more economically. Although implementing a speaker system throughout a 15-story high-rise building may require a substantial monetary investment, the institution could use the built-in paging system with the phone service, if the phones are installed using voice-over Internet protocol (VOIP), such as the system implemented at DePaul University in Chicago, Illinois (DePaul University, 2014).

Because all buildings are required to have fire alarm systems, many times PAs can be installed using the existing speakers connected to a computer program. Regardless of the mechanism and type of campus, it is imperative that there is an audible alert system, to not only inform those who did not sign up for text alerts but also inform campus visitors and faculty who may be teaching where phones are turned off or on silent.

In a chapter about technology use in a campus crisis, Mastrodicasa (2008) reviewed communication with new technology, such as e-mail, text messaging, and social networking sites, such as Facebook. As the technology options have evolved, numerous new communication methods have appeared, others have dissipated, and all are used at varying rates. While options discussed in this text were viable at the time of writing, they may not remain so ongoing. The rapid shift in communication preferences must be monitored on each college campus in order to remain effective, but social media channels remain an important part of disseminating information. At the same time, social media can be a haven for misinformation; building redundancy into the notification system means that multiple methods, including official, familiar channels, such as e-mail, are also utilized.

The notification of the Virginia Tech shooting was initially sent to students by e-mail. Although e-mail is instantly dispersed, the communication strategy was widely criticized for its slow notification to the campus community, as most students did not actually check their e-mail and receive the information (Mastrodicasa, 2008). Accordingly, it was determined that Virginia Tech did not provide a timely warning as required by the Clery Act (Clery Center, 2014). As a result, many campuses adopted various instant alert systems using text messaging to provide communication that students could receive immediately (Gow, McGee, Townsend, Anderson, & Varnhagen, 2009; Haddow & Haddow, 2014; Mastrodicasa, 2008).

Gow et al. (2009) provided a review of emergency alert options for college campuses, primarily featuring the emergency alert text as one method to be used in conjunction with multiple communication methods, and how it would be viewed by college students. West and Valentini (2013) noted that over the past decade, campuses have made significant investments in mass notification systems with multiple layers of necessary redundancy, such as digital signage in classrooms and meeting areas, indoor and outdoor sirens, messaging via social media outlets, computer pop-ups, and wireless alerts (West & Valentini, 2013). For example, Florida State University has approximately 25 different types of communication used for safety notifications (Negrea, 2014). In 2014, campus shooting incidents, such as at Seattle Pacific University, still triggered emergency alert text messages and e-mail messages to warn students (Jaschik, 2014). Although text messaging is certainly a quick method of notifying students, some campus officials suggest that students are not reacting with concern to the information as they should due to the frequency of the texts (Misner, 2014).

The fact that college students have nearly constant access to the Internet through either a smartphone or laptop has changed the way adults manage decisions. In 2012, some 70% of all cell phone owners and 86% of smartphone owners reported using their phones in the previous 30 days to solve a "just-in-time" issue, such as handling an unexpected problem, finding information, or settling a dispute, and 19% even used it to get help in an emergency situation (Rainie & Fox, 2012). Younger cell phone users are more likely than older users to have utilized smartphones in such a manner; 88% of cell phone owners ages 18–29 performed one of these just-in-time activities in the past 30 days (Rainie & Fox, 2012).

Social Media and Two-way Communication

The important thing to remember is that communication during a crisis cannot, and should not, be one-way. That is to say, faculty, staff, and students must be able to inform campus safety and/or members of the CMT that there is an incident developing. All too often, the assumption is that the crisis responders will know about the situation and inform members of the campus community. Unfortunately, that is idealistic and, perhaps, unrealistic. It is more likely that the situation will develop in a classroom or common space and community members will need to alert the authorities. Some campuses, such as Gulf Coast State, have installed panic buttons in classrooms and common spaces that, if activated, alert campus police via a mobile app to where the incident is occurring (Bolkan, 2013).

Primarily, colleges and universities must remember that whereas they have limited control over the outbreak of a crisis situation, they *do* have control over how they respond before, during, and after the event. Accordingly, the onus will be on the institution to communicate regularly and effectively during a crisis or emergency situation in as many ways as possible. To that end, technology and preprinted materials are good in theory, but they are useless if there are not adequate numbers of people trained, cross-trained, and appointed to use said systems when a crisis develops. The PIO on the CMT is responsible for ensuring there is a subcommittee that includes the frontline security personnel and student affairs on-call staff who understand how to send out messages and craft the content of those messages. The team as a whole must ensure that the precrisis announcements prepare everyone for what may occur.

Emergency management applications for mobile devices have drastically increased as more people rely on those mobile devices for instant and accurate information (Haddow & Haddow, 2014; O'Neil, 2014; Todd, 2013; West & Valentini, 2013). West and Valentini (2013) cite the international disasters of the Haitian earthquake in 2010 and the Japanese tsunami in 2011 as examples in which mobile technology became crucial to the response and recovery. In the United States, several universities have begun using mobile platforms for a wide range of activities, including emergency communications (Haddow & Haddow, 2014; Negrea, 2014; O'Neil, 2014; Todd, 2013; West & Valentini, 2013). As of 2013, 79% of colleges and universities planned to activate, or have already activated, mobile apps (Negrea, 2014). Similarly, the rise of mobile apps for cell phones and tablets has created an environment in which community members can report a concern to authorities immediately, without the implementation of "blue phones" around campus. Community members can also research various resources to solve problems, such as first aid needs or where a shelter might be (Negrea, 2014). The ideas for apps range from more individualized ones, where people can set up a network to notify authorities if they have not reached their destination in a certain amount of time, to immediate alerts to campus safety personnel ("Personal Safety," 2011). The challenge with implementing these systems is that if not monitored they create a greater liability for the institution. In short, having no system is better than having a system that is not properly implemented, thereby creating a false sense of security.

Currently, there is much debate regarding the best approach for utilizing mobile apps, and several companies are developing apps (in addition to homegrown systems). Although specific features vary, many of the new apps create a two-way channel of communication, with written or visual messages tagged with their GPS location, with public-safety officials, who can respond to alerts with follow-up questions or specific instructions (O'Neil, 2014; Todd, 2013). For example, LiveSafe connects students and campus police in a two-way dialogue via their smartphones, Pathlight at the University of Chicago lets students opt into GPS tracking services, and Northwestern State University's app allows users to opt in to a feature that communicates to police where they are going and when they should arrive (O'Neil, 2014; West & Valentini, 2013).

When a university uses an opt-in system, it cannot rely on that communication tool alone to notify individuals. For example, the University of Alberta decided not include an emergency button on its My UAlberta app because it would have required more steps than to simply dial 911 (Negrea, 2014). Instead, the University of Alberta uses its app to send weather and emergency alerts to anyone who has opted into the system, which provides an even faster route of instant communication than text messaging (Negrea, 2014). Similarly, about 25% of Florida State University's student body has not downloaded the Florida State University mobile app, and emergency alerts are instead sent by text message (Negrea, 2014). Experts state that campuses should use multiple methods to contact students to be most effective (Misner, 2014).

Zuckerman (2014) suggests five items for campuses to consider when deciding upon a mobile safety application:

1. Features most relevant to your campus
2. Integration
3. Clery Act compliance
4. Ease of use and setup
5. Cost

Beyond official campus communication, mobile technology plays a role in how individuals communicate with each other during a campus crisis. For example, during campus shootings at both Virginia Tech in 2007 and Northern Illinois University in 2008, individuals used mobile technology to communicate with others and to give real-time updates regarding the events as they unfolded (Haddow & Haddow, 2014). Additionally, they used Facebook and other social media to interact with others, seek information about the incidents, share experiences, develop online relationships, and build community awareness of the events (Haddow & Haddow, 2014). There are several apps that provide a way for individuals to connect with each other after such an incident, find shelter, learn basic first aid information, and more (Haddow & Haddow, 2014; Negrea, 2014).

A full day before traditional media compiled a list, all 32 of the victims of the Virginia Tech shooting had been identified through information posted by students on Facebook (Haddow & Haddow, 2014). Similarly, the 2013 Boston Marathon bombings were first reported on Facebook and Twitter, and slightly more than half of young adults 18–29 years old received bombing-related news via social media (Haddow & Haddow, 2014). Haddow and Haddow (2014) state that they expect the use of digital media during disasters to continue to skyrocket as the use of the technology increases.

In preparing your own campus for using social media during an emergency response, it is important to remember that having set response messages is key. These templates should be simple and factual and convey consistency. It is quite easy to fall into the social media trap of responding with a terse note or ambiguous comment. That will not prove fruitful in the end. Use social media to take in necessary information but convey a consistent message.

Putting Theory Into Practice

In today's high-tech environment, responding quickly to an active shooter is paramount. Administrators must be mindful of having the appropriate technology or communication system in place to ensure a timely response. This section attempts to move beyond theory by analyzing real-world incidents.

Shooting at the University of Texas

In September 2010, a sophomore at the University of Texas brought an AK-47 to campus, randomly fired shots into the ground, ran into the library, and turned the gun on himself. The first report was made to 911 at 8:12 a.m., and the campus sent a text alert at 8:19 a.m., saying that an armed subject was last seen at the campus library. At 8:25 a.m. the campus siren was activated and loudspeaker announcements were provided every 10 minutes (Corley & Latham, 2011).

There was a social media post at 8:30 a.m., a campuswide e-mail at 8:37 a.m., and a posting on the emergency website at 8:37 a.m. (Corley & Latham, 2011). At 8:41 a.m., the instructions to shelter in place went out via text message and social media (Corley & Latham, 2011).

In the analysis of the communication of the incident, Corley and Latham (2011) indicated the success of reaching 51,000 students and 24,000 faculty and staff quickly by preparing message templates for all scenarios, having an emergency plan in place, setting up redundancies, and aligning the emergency management page with the university's home page for maximum impact. They also discussed the challenges of social media in such an incident; specifically, they recommended disabling comments and making Facebook a one-way communication tool during such events and informing the campus community about what has happened (Corley & Latham, 2011). They identified several challenges, including cell phones dying and the terms *lockdown*, *shelter in place*, and *suspect* not resonating with the audience; it was necessary to report updates every 15–20 minutes—if only to communicate that there was no new information (Corley & Latham, 2011). There were many requests for public records after the event, and the authors recommended documenting feeds, web, and social media channels immediately (Corley & Latham, 2011).

Lone Star College–North Harris Campus Shooting

In January 2013, a shooting incident on a 19,000-student campus located in the outskirts of Houston occurred in which two male students were in a dispute. Three people were injured ("Shooting," 2014). Administrators were able to secure a lockdown on campus, but they found that their communications channels were unprepared to deal with the large volume of cellular traffic, and text messaging was delayed by 20 minutes ("Shooting," 2014). Additionally, it was not until the incident occurred that administrators realized 400,000 names had accumulated in their emergency texting system over the years, and many of those needed to be deleted once they were no longer part of the immediate campus community ("Shooting," 2014). They also recommended considering the various constituencies within a campus community that might need special communications—such as Spanish speakers, nontraditional-aged students, D/deaf students—and having a plan to reach them ("Shooting," 2014).

University of Central Florida Incident

In March 2013, a student committed suicide with a gun in the residence hall at the University of Central Florida, but within hours of his death, law enforcement officers investigating the scene discovered hundreds of rounds of ammunition, an assault weapon, homemade explosives, and a plan-to-kill "to-do" list, as well as a plan to injure as many University of Central Florida students as possible (University of Central Florida, 2013). The review of the incident found that the emergency alerts sent by text and e-mail were well managed; Facebook and Twitter were effectively utilized to communicate important updates, correct misinformation circulating online, and connect students, employees, parents, media, and others to assistance resources (University of Central Florida, 2013). Areas of concern were the capabilities and effectiveness of the UCF emergency alert process and whether students' families and all employees should be added into the alert system, making it even larger than the 70,000 campus stakeholders currently listed within the system, as well as looking ahead at the intended campus growth (University of Central Florida, 2013).

University of Rhode Island Gun on Campus

In April 2013, a report of an individual with a gun in a large lecture hall of approximately 300 students was made to campus police at the University of Rhode Island at 11:19 a.m. (University of Rhode Island, 2013). After police cleared the building and no shooter was discovered, they were not able to send an emergency alert until 11:50 a.m.; a campus alert on the blue phones went out at 11:58 a.m. (University of Rhode Island, 2013). A review indicated that they needed to constantly prepare for such emergencies, including reducing the number of approvals required prior to disseminating the emergency message; increasing the frequency of notifications, even if only to reiterate that there was no new information; increasing the number of individuals registered with the emergency alert system from

80%; and having an emergency home page template to use to reduce server load (University of Rhode Island, 2013).

Boston Marathon Bombing

In April 2013, two bombs exploded at the end of the Boston Marathon, and several Boston-area college campuses were impacted as members of their campus communities were attending the event and running in the marathon; a graduate student and a campus public safety officer from two different campuses were killed (Milstone, 2014). As the investigation progressed, it was determined that the person sought for the bombing was a student at the University of Massachusetts–Dartmouth. Campus text and e-mail alerts were sent to faculty, staff, and students, telling them to remain in their current locations and informing others to remain off campus (Milstone, 2014). Instructions were posted on the UMass–Dartmouth website, call centers were staffed and remained open in the president's and student affairs offices, and the entire campus was eventually evacuated (Milstone, 2014). Managing the evacuation communications and logistics required specific focus and planning (Milstone, 2014). Milstone (2014) states that the media were critical of the campus regarding the lack of information about the student in question, and the failure to release federally protected educational records; subsequently, there were accusations that the university had harbored a terrorist. The importance of communication simply cannot be overstated. Communication strategies used during the Boston Marathon bombing were identified as successful and included frequent updating of web postings, the campus alert system, and phone communication staffing by experienced individuals who had accurate and updated information (Milstone, 2014).

Shooting at Seattle Pacific University

In June 2014, a nonstudent allegedly walked into an academic building on the campus of Seattle Pacific University (SPU), a small Christian college in Seattle, armed with a shotgun, and shot three people, killing one before pausing to reload his weapon. During this brief span of time, a student hired by the campus as a building monitor used pepper spray to stop the assailant; several bystanders then helped him to restrain the shooter before authorities arrived (Rigby, 2014). SPU's Crisis Management webpage provides specific information to faculty, staff, and students as to what to do in a crisis and provides that information in each classroom, in addition to appointing building emergency coordinators (BECs), who know what to do in times of crisis (Seattle Pacific University, 2014a). In the aftermath of the incident, SPU provided a dedicated page for resources, as well as a page on social media for members to share information and for the institution to respond accordingly (Seattle Pacific University, 2014b).

Conclusion

The importance of having an emergency plan, practicing and testing the systems, and having the communications strategy prepared has been reiterated throughout this chapter. The changing nature of how the campus community, especially college students, communicates must be taken into consideration as plans are developed. The campus community must be supplied with frequent updates via text, social media, and websites, even if there is nothing new to report. Knowing that most adults on a campus community have access to a smartphone adds an additional layer of demand for instant information. Campuses should rehearse emergency exercises and have prepared messaging scenarios to make notifications as quickly as possible without having to draft the details. Each incident at any college campus provides lessons for improving preparation for potential future incidents.

References

Bolkan, J. (2013, September 11). Gulf Coast State College deploys panic buttons for emergency response. *Campus Technology*. Retrieved from http://campustechnology .com/articles/2013/09/11/gulf-coast-state-college-deploys-panic-buttons-for-emergency-response.aspx

Carter, S. D. (n.d.). Timely warning vs. emergency notification: What's the big difference? *Campus Safety Magazine*. Retrieved from http://www.campussafetymagazine .com/article/timely-warnings-vs-emergency-notifications-what-s-the-big-difference

Clery Center for Security on Campus. (2014). *Summary of the Jeanne Clery Act.* Retrieved from http://clerycenter.org/summary-jeanne-clery-act

Corley, N., & Latham, C. (2011, October). *Crisis communication on the web.* Paper presented at Higher Ed Web Conference, Austin, TX.

Dahlstrom, E., Walker, J. D., & Dziuban, C. (2013). *ECAR study of undergraduate students and information technology.* Louisville, CO: EDUCAUSE Center for Analysis and Research. Retrieved from www.educause.edu/library/resources/ecar-study-undergraduate-students-and-information-technology-2013

DePaul University. (2014). *DePaul University emergency operations plan.* Retrieved from https://emergencyplan.depaul.edu

Duggan, M., & Smith, A. (2013, December 30). *Social media update 2013.* Washington, DC: Pew Research Center. Retrieved from http://pewinternet.org/Reports/2013/Social-Media-Update.aspx

Facebook. (2014). *Company info.* Retrieved from http://newsroom.fb.com/company-info

Gow, G. A., McGee, T., Townsend, D., Anderson, P., & Varnhagen, S. (2009, Summer). Communication technology, emergency alerts, and campus safety. *IEEE Technology and Society Magazine, 28*(2), 34–41.

Haddow, G. D., & Haddow, K. S. (2014). *Disaster communications in a changing media world* (2nd ed.). Waltham, MA: Elsevier.

Harper, K. S., Paterson, B. G., & Zdziarski, G. L. (Eds.). (2006). *Crisis management: Responding from the heart.* Washington, DC: NASPA.

Homeland Security presidential directive-5. (2003, February 28). Retrieved from https://www.dhs.gov/sites/default/files/publications/Homeland%20Security%20Presidential%20Directive%205.pdf

Jaschik, S. (2013, October 21). Texting in class. *Inside Higher Ed.* Retrieved from http://www.insidehighered.com/news/2013/10/21/study-documents-how-much-students-text-during-class#sthash.qsurxOwB.dpbs

Jaschik, S. (2014, June 6). Another deadly shooting. *Inside Higher Ed.* Retrieved from http://www.insidehighered.com/news/2014/06/06/shooter-kills-one-injures-others-seattle-pacific-u#sthash.xQDVVTLO.aEcuHY5W.dpbs

Junco, R. (2013). Inequalities in Facebook use. *Computers in Human Behavior, 29*(6), 2328–2336.

Junco, R., & Cole-Avent, G. (2008). An introduction to technologies commonly used by college students. In R. Junco & D. M. Timm (Eds.), *Using emerging technologies to enhance student engagement* (pp. 3–17). New Directions for Student Services, no. 124 (special issue). San Francisco, CA: Wiley Periodicals.

Junco, R., & Mastrodicasa, J. (2007). *Connecting to the net.generation: What higher education professionals need to know about today's students.* Washington, DC: NASPA.

Junco, R., Merson, D., & Salter, D. W. (2010). The effect of gender, ethnicity, and income on college students' use of communication technologies. *Cyberpsychology, Behavior, and Social Networking, 13*(6), 619–627.

Kolowich, S. (2011, January 6). How will students communicate? *Inside Higher Ed.* Retrieved from http://www.insidehighered.com/news/2011/01/06/college_technology_officers_consider_changing_norms_in_student_communications #sthash.Oug7BSFG.dpbs

Kolowich, S. (2012, October 22). Outsourcing privacy. *Inside Higher Ed*. Retrieved from http://www.insidehighered.com/news/2012/10/22/universities-and-microsoft-write-standard-privacy-agreement-cloud-services#sthash.bTcAFwfS.dpbs

Lawson, C. J. (2007). Crisis communication. In E. L. Zdziarski, N. W. Dunkel, J. M. Rollo, & associates (Eds.), *Campus crisis management: A comprehensive guide to planning, prevention, response, and recovery* (pp. 97–120). San Francisco, CA: Jossey-Bass.

Mastrodicasa, J. (2008). Technology use in campus crisis. In R. Junco & D. M. Timm (Eds.), *Using emerging technologies to enhance student engagement* (pp. 37–53). New Directions for Student Services, no. 124 (special issue). San Francisco, CA: Wiley Periodicals.

Mastrodicasa, J., & Metellus, P. (2013, February). The impact of social media on college students. *Journal of College and Character, 14*(1), 21–30.

McCoy, B. (2013, October). Digital distractions in the classroom: Student classroom use of digital devices for non-class related purposes. *Journal of Media Education, 4*(4), 5–14.

Milstone, D. (2014, Winter). When the world is watching: Lessons learned in dealing with campus crises. *NASPA Leadership Exchange*, 20–22.

Misner, J. (2014, September 19). Too many campus alerts? Officials worry that students increasingly tune them out. *The Chronicle of Higher Education*. Retrieved from http://chronicle.com/article/Too-Many-Campus-Alerts-/148897

Negrea, S. (2014, July). Apps move up. *University Business*, 41–43.

O'Neil, M. (2014, March 10). Sophisticated mobile apps are shaping campus safety. *The Chronicle of Higher Education*. Retrieved from http://chronicle.com/article/Sophisticated-Mobile-Apps-Are/145151/

Personal safety apps: The next generation of blue light phones. (2011, September 26). *Campus Safety Magazine*. Retrieved from http://www.campussafetymagazine.com/article/Personal-Safety-Apps-The-Next-Generation-of-Blue-Light-Phones

Pew Research Center. (2014, January). *Mobile technology fact sheet*. Retrieved from http://www.pewinternet.org/fact-sheets/mobile-technology-fact-sheet

Rainie, L., & Fox, S. (2012, May 7). *Just-in-time information through mobile connections*. Retrieved from http://www.pewinternet.org/2012/05/07/just-in-time-information-through-mobile-connections

Rigby, B. (2014, June 6). Accused Seattle gunman suffers severe mental illness, his lawyer says. *Reuters*. Retrieved from http://www.reuters.com/article/2014/06/06/us-usa-shooting-seattle-idUSKBN0EH11D20140606

Rollo, M., & Zdziarski, E. L. (2007). The impact of crisis. In E. L. Zdziarski, N. W. Dunkel, J. M. Rollo, & associates (Eds.), *Campus crisis management: A comprehensive guide to planning, prevention, response, and recovery* (pp. 3–34). San Francisco, CA: Jossey-Bass.

Rubin, C. (2013, September 27). Technology and the college generation. *New York Times*, p. ST2.

Seattle Pacific University. (2014a). *Emergency plan*. Retrieved from http://spu.edu/about-spu/press-room/emergency-plan

Seattle Pacific University. (2014b). *Recovery information*. Retrieved from http://www.spu.edu/about-spu/press-room/emergency-plan/spu-recovery-information

Shooting rocks Lone Star College campus. (2014, Winter). *NASPA Leadership Exchange*, p. 24. Retreived from http://www.leadershipexchange-digital.com/lead ershipexchange/2014winter?pg=26#pg26

Todd, D. M. (2013, April 19). Local colleges use advanced technology to warn students about campus emergencies. *Pittsburgh Post-Gazette*. Retrieved from http://www.post-gazette.com/businessnews/2013/04/19/Local-colleges-use-advanced-technology-to-warn-students-about-campus-emergencies/stories/201304190134

Twitter. (2014). *About*. Retrieved from https://about.twitter.com/company

University of Central Florida. (2013, May 31). *UCF after-action review*. Retrieved from https://www.llis.dhs.gov/sites/default/files/UCF%20Tower%20Shooting%20 AAR-IP.pdf

University of Rhode Island. (2013, April 29). *Chafee Social Science Center incident report*. Retrieved from www.uri.edu/emergency/ChafeeApril2013.pdf

West, D. M., & Valentini, E. (2013, July 16). *How mobile devices are transforming disaster relief and public safety*. Washington, DC: Brookings Institution. Retrieved from http://www.brookings.edu/research/papers/2013/07/16-mobile-technology-disaster-relief-west

Zuckerman, J. (2014, May 16). 5 tips to help your campus select a mobile security solution. *Campus Safety Magazine*. Retrieved from http://www.campussafety magazine.com/article/5_tips_to_help_your_campus_select_a_mobile_security _solution

8 A Small-College Perspective

Steve Jacobson and Sheila Lambert

IN RECENT years, colleges and universities within the United States have focused on increasing campus safety and keeping their students, faculty, and staff safe from violence. Violence often manifests itself in a variety of ways, including, but not limited to, incidents involving domestic abuse, sexual assault, bullying, and gun violence. Incidents of gun violence, in particular, have received increased attention from the media and within student affairs due to the size and scope of many recent campus tragedies. These incidents occur on campuses regardless of location, mission, or size and have been seen at both public and private large universities, as well as smaller, regionally based institutions. Although smaller institutions (those with an undergraduate population of fewer than 5,000) have often been successful in offering personalized student educational experiences, they are faced with unique challenges that larger public and private institutions do not experience. Because there are over 4,000 colleges and universities within the United States, it is imperative to consider how these institutions are addressing such challenges, preparing their campuses for gun-related violence, and identifying the best practices to prevent violence from occurring (U.S. Department of Education, Office of Safe and Drug-Free Schools, 2010).

Many small colleges and universities face limitations in funding, resources, and staff. Despite these challenges, they are able to successfully change their campus and community cultures by responding to changing legislation through the development of comprehensive, intentional, and systematic gun violence prevention initiatives. This chapter explores two successful small-college violence prevention programs, reviews best practices for violence prevention, and offers recommendations about how small colleges and universities can create an impact within their campus and their community.

Gun Violence and the Campus Landscape

Looking back over the last 2 decades, it would have been difficult to believe permitting guns on a college or university campus would even be considered. "Yet by 2012, guns were allowed on 200 public campuses in six states. That number appears certain to increase; in 2011 alone, bills to permit guns on campus were introduced in 23 state legislatures" (Birnbaum, 2013). With the increase in the number of guns appearing on campus, there has been a parallel increase in the amount of violent, gun-related incidents. Birnbaum (2013) recently reported that

> [T]he Secret Service, the Office of Education, and the FBI (Drysdale, Modzeleski, & Simons, 2010) analyzed 272 incidents of targeted violence on college campuses that occurred between 1990 and 2008. Guns were used in 54 percent of the reported cases, and almost 60 percent of fatal violent incidents were instigated against someone previously known to the assailant.

In addition, the U.S. Department of Education in 2008 found that college campuses within the United States had over 2,100 arrests for illegal weapons, over 24,000 arrests for illicit drugs, over 31,000 arrests for burglary, and over 50 arrests for murder (U.S. Department of Education, 2014). These incidents are in addition to any student conduct violations that may have been adjudicated through institutional judicial processes and did not involve the legal system.

To be clear, even though the number of gun-related violence issues has risen, it is not just a college or university phenomenon. Gun violence is a greater societal issue that is now manifesting itself on the college campus. As a society, regardless of one's interpretation of rights awarded to citizens by the U.S. Constitution to bear arms, we must all take a stand to prevent gun-related incidents from occurring in the first place. For society to address this issue it must focus on the underlying conditions and causes, including, but not limited to, lack of parental involvement, limited access to mentors, and increased gun activity. As part of this review, it is important to understand the small-college landscape and its challenges in fully implementing gun violence prevention strategies.

Changing Demographics

A demographic shift has been occurring in the types and numbers of students attending college. This change includes an increasing number of students who choose to delay their attendance. Fewer traditional-aged students (18–22 years of age) are attending smaller colleges and universities now that the "baby boom echo" has peaked. Additionally, small colleges are seeing an increasing number of students from marginalized populations, veteran and military students, and students who also have a family (Luzer, 2013). All of these factors are challenging institutions, especially those that are smaller and tuition driven, to change their recruitment, retention, and graduation attainment programs and services. Although many of these educational programs, including those that focus on gun violence prevention, may have worked in the past, they may not work well with today's students and those in future generations.

Increasing Costs

With tuition costs continuing to rise, students and families are asking why it is important to take on a large expense without a clear assurance that they will obtain a career in their chosen field and be able to pay off their large student debt (Marklein, 2013). For many small, tuition-driven institutions, the days of simply increasing tuition to implement new academic majors and important new programs are over. Many small institutions have faced budget cuts due to either lower enrollments or the need to reorganize financial resources in order to create new academic programs that attract additional students. This means fewer resources for new "nonacademic" programs.

Increasing Competition

In addition to curbing tuition increases, smaller colleges are experiencing increased competition. Whereas some institutions have faced difficult recruitment challenges for many years, the rise of for-profit and online colleges has forced colleges and universities to develop new teaching formats. These formats are different from the traditional, lecture-based educational models and are aimed at meeting the needs of millennial and nontraditional students. These changes have also led institutions to focus less on cocurricular programs and more on those academic programs and majors that recruit students (Selingo, 2013). This significantly limits the resources allocated to other equally important issues, such as violence prevention.

Staffing and Resource Limitations

Because many small colleges and universities are tuition dependent and have smaller endowments, some may face a lack of staffing and resources. Although many of these institutions focus on being student centered by offering small class environments and having direct student access to faculty and staff, they are increasingly challenged to offer a superior learning environment with shrinking budgets and increasing layoffs of administrative staff, especially after the recession of 2008. It is only recently that institutions began considering adding staff positions and restoring programs that were previously cut (Kiley, 2012).

Unfunded Federal Mandates

As a requirement of accepting federal financial aid funds, the U.S. government has increasingly placed more requirements upon colleges and universities. Often in response to public demand, these requirements are frequently unfunded, leaving it to institutions to find financial resources and staff to fulfill the requirements. Many large colleges and universities possess adequate staffing or have the ability to hire additional staff, making it easier to meet federal requirements. At smaller institutions this proves to be an increasing challenge, especially if enrollment is stagnant or falling, as tuition barely covers costs and the endowment is unable to support the institution. This ultimately leads to existing faculty and staff having to take on additional roles and responsibilities. As a result, many small institutions offer only the essential programs and services required by law, leaving other important services unavailable to students. This leads to programs being neither fully executed nor meeting overall intentions and mandates (e.g., enforcing drug laws on campus, Title IX issues).

Family Demands

As the children of Generation X arrive on campus, colleges and universities have found that families play a significant role in their students' lives (English, 2013). Family members are an integral part of the college decision-making process; they have clear expectations and demands about their student's safety while at college. These demands have included requiring institutions to prevent sexual assault and address sexual misconduct between students, including upholding students' rights during student conduct hearings for complainants and respondents alike. Although many institutions have implemented tools to respond to these demands (e.g., increased camera usage, enhanced police patrols on and off campus, university emergency notification systems, updated crisis response plans), more is being asked of institutions to prevent violence on campus.

Best Policies and Practices

Regardless of a college's location and size, violence can and does affect everyone. For institutions of higher education, it is imperative to create safe, violence-free campuses and build relationships that foster proactive results. In order to accomplish these goals, universities (especially small institutions) must develop collaborative partnerships across the academy and design programs that will meet the needs of both the on- and off-campus communities. The challenge for a small college is developing and implementing plans with limited funds and resources. Several suggestions for successful policies and practices that have worked on small campuses are highlighted here:

- ➤ Policies
  - ➤ Develop clear and well-communicated on-campus gun policies. Because some states are now requiring their public institutions to permit students and staff to carry weapons on-campus, policies must be written that uphold the law, but also protect the members of the community. If a campus prohibits guns on campus, the institution must strictly enforce its policy and offer serious consequences. (J. Winn, personal communication, June 6, 2014)

- ➤ Practices
  - ➤ Threat assessment teams should be established and regularly meet. This multidisciplinary team should be designed to assess concerning student behavior and set up a system to perform early actions and interventions. The team should consist of a variety of campus partners, including public safety, residence life, student conduct, academic advising,

faculty, wellness/counseling, and other key departments within the institution.

> The college or university should conduct weekly judicial team meetings and conduct meetings with key stakeholders to review current student behavior.

> Faculty, staff, and student training should be offered on campus regarding how to detect concerning or threatening behavior and how to refer a student directly or anonymously.

> Strong collaboration with the university counseling center must be maintained so mental health assessments and interventions can be implemented and students who need additional mental health services can be monitored and/or referred to local hospitals or providers.

> Emergency backup contracts with area mental health agencies and positive working relationships with community mental health agencies must be fostered to ensure collaborative working relationships.

> A strong, positive relationship with local police and first responders who are aware of the university policies and emergency management systems is essential to protecting the campus community.

> Institutions must offer parents education about mental health issues and how to deal with a concern about their student. Sharing information about how to refer their student for service or assessment is critical. (J. Winn, personal communication, June 6, 2014)

Educational Programs

In an effort to ensure everyone is aware of the policies and standards, strong and continuous education about university conduct and gun policies on campus must be offered to students, faculty, and staff. One educational resource that has proven helpful to many small colleges is the Enough Is Enough antiviolence campaign. An offering of NASPA–Student Affairs Administrators in Higher Education, this campaign is designed to create a new paradigm for peace and safety and was founded after the tragic events that occurred at the Virginia Polytechnic Institute and State University (Virginia Tech) on April

16, 2007. The program aims to address societal violence through three main areas of focus: a nationwide prevention and intervention campaign, legislative efforts, and the provision of resources. The campaign's goal is to establish an Enough Is Enough cross-disciplinary committee on each campus, aimed at working together toward establishing comprehensive, intentional, and systematic violence prevention initiatives. This type of campaign encourages the entire campus to take action by reporting concerning behavior and creating a safe environment.

Many small universities are incorporating strong violence prevention programs on their campuses and have made a tremendous impact in their communities. Two such schools are University of the Pacific (Pacific), located in Stockton, California, and Southern New Hampshire University (SNHU), in Manchester, New Hampshire. Both Pacific and SNHU were named National Model Schools with NASPA's Enough Is Enough campaign and have excelled in offering programs and services that work to prevent gun violence.

University of the Pacific

Pacific's Enough Is Enough campaign is a multifaceted program designed to educate students about the impact of violence and to serve as a "call to action" for the community to collectively develop innovative violence reduction strategies. In order to create a comprehensive initiative, a committee of faculty, staff, students, and community partners came together and focused on three key dimensions for programming and strategy development: Pacific's Stockton campus, K–12 colleagues, and community partners. Through these three areas, Pacific's Enough Is Enough campaign emphasizes five learning outcomes. These learning outcomes are that students be able to:

1. identify the key messages of the Pacific Enough Is Enough campaign program in which they participated;
2. recognize agencies and organizations within the Stockton community that work to reduce violence;
3. identify a specific action or strategy that students can employ to reduce violence within the community;
4. seek out ways to be involved in violence prevention efforts; and
5. engage and participate in interventions to reduce violence.

Pacific hosted a variety of campus programs during the national Enough Is Enough Week held during the first week of April. These programs focused on the core causes of violence (as opposed to symptoms) and included themes each day of the week, including Breaking the Chains of Violence and Poverty; Violence as a Public Health Issue; and Be the Change, Make a Difference. The programs for the week included an antiviolence art show, speakers who focused on preventing domestic abuse and sexual assault, presentations by community partners and organizations, and a program discussing what has happened in the 20 years since a tragic shooting at the local Cleveland Elementary School (Richman & Emmons, 2014). The week was highlighted by the Enough Is Enough Hero's Award reception, where the university recognized key individuals and organizations that have made significant contributions to reducing violence within the San Joaquin Valley. The ceremony featured Gwen Dungy, past NASPA executive director, as the keynote speaker. At the conclusion of the Enough Is Enough Week, students were asked to pledge to reduce violence and take the initiative to make a difference within their community. These pledges were then made into a collage and hung prominently in the University Center. All events were assessed to determine if the learning outcomes were met.

Pacific selected Cleveland Elementary as a campaign partner and worked with the school's administration, faculty, and students to support a variety of programs. These programs included the Cleveland University Bound Scholars (CUBS), which aims to enhance students' social and emotional skills; a mentorship and academic tutoring program; and a structured recess program to reduce bullying. Cleveland students and families were also invited to a Pacific baseball game that not only focused on the connection that Cleveland has with Pacific (a Cleveland student was asked to throw the first pitch) but also encouraged reading skills improvement with books donated by Barnes & Noble. Due to Pacific's involvement with the school, Cleveland changed its mascot to a tiger cub, reflective of Pacific's tiger mascot, and the school colors to orange and black.

Due to the strong town/gown relationship Pacific has with the surrounding community, the Enough Is Enough committee developed several connections with local agencies and developed Enough Is Enough internships. These semester internships were structured so students received academic credit for their work with community agencies whose mission relates to reducing violence. In addition, students were able to "skip a meal" in order to raise funds for a local violence prevention community agency. The university's food service vendor, Bon Appetit, enabled Pacific students to donate over $2,000 for the Women's Center of San Joaquin.

Assessment data for the campaign came from multiple sources, including institutional data, student participant rates, and comments/reports. The assessment plan for this initiative was both formative and summative, addressing immediate outcomes and longer-term impacts. Overarching learning goals included increased awareness of localized issues and origins of violence and engagement with systemic solutions through active community partnerships. Ultimately, the longitudinal indicator for the success of this initiative showed an overall reduction in activities that demonstrate disregard and disrespect for others that could result in violent actions, increased awareness of the Enough Is Enough campaign and localized issues of violence and their origins, and increased leadership capacity of a targeted group of Pacific students to impact school-based violence.

Southern New Hampshire University

SNHU established its Enough Is Enough campaign initiative in January 2011. Upon inception, SNHU created a standing universitywide committee that represented key departments in both student and academic affairs. This group met and developed a strategic plan to coordinate the university's violence prevention efforts and include them in the Enough Is Enough campaign. The outcomes for the campaign included:

- train students, faculty, and staff on bystander intervention;
- create a safe environment that shares a culture of respect;
- collaborate with communitywide departments on all violence-related events; and
- develop an Enough Is Enough logo, create advertisements with Enough Is Enough messages, and purchase promotional materials that include Enough Is Enough messages.

SNHU's Enough Is Enough committee decided to implement the campaign through a multiyear plan. Each year builds upon the success of the previous year. The campaign began in 2011 with marketing and branding efforts that included the following:

> *Creating a campus logo.* The committee developed a university-specific logo designed around the national logo for the Enough Is Enough campaign in order to establish a clear identity in the community.
> *Filming an Enough Is Enough video.* The committee wrote a script for a video and contacted students, faculty, and staff to ask for participation. Those participating in the video included president Paul LeBlanc, then vice president of student affairs Scott Kalicki, Heather Lorenz (currently the dean of students), athletes, students with disabilities, fraternity and sorority members, student leaders, students of color, and so on. The Enough Is Enough video was produced and edited by an SNHU student and presented in multiple venues on campus, including on the TV screen at the entrance to the dining hall. Additionally, students signed a pledge to refrain from acts of violence.
> *Developing programs.* Numerous events were planned and highlighted the video and opportunity to take the pledge to prevent violence. Resident assistants were trained in bystander intervention, the public safety office held a women's safety clinic, a sorority kicked off the clothesline project, and fraternities and athletic teams participated in a white ribbon campaign.
> *Organizing giveaways.* Shirts with the Enough Is Enough logo were distributed to committee members and used as giveaways for events. Whistles and safety flashlights with the campaign logo were distributed at all events, helping to educate the community about the antiviolence campaign.

Once the committee assessed the progress of the previous 6 months, it decided to introduce the Enough Is Enough campaign as a yearlong initiative. After learning several departments at the university were already holding violence prevention programs, leadership determined that all antiviolence programs should fall under the umbrella of the Enough Is Enough campaign. As a result, the campaign was able to include, coordinate, and highlight a variety of important violence prevention events throughout the 2011–2012 academic year. These initiatives included the following:

➤ *Take Back the Night*. This national event raises awareness of sexual assault and asks community members to walk in support of all those affected by sexual assault. The event drew many community members and was attended by 300 students, faculty, and staff. Enough Is Enough campaign materials were distributed at this event. The committee created a slide show as a spring kickoff event.

➤ *Kickoff week*. The kickoff week included a second video, highlighting Enough Is Enough events from the previous year. The video was shown in multiple venues, where students were given the opportunity to sign the Enough Is Enough pledge. Hundreds of signatures were collected as the effort continued to teach people to prevent violence.

➤ *Partnering with athletics*. During the month of February, the Enough Is Enough committee brought the pledge to a women's basketball game and a men's hockey game. The pledge was available for the public to sign, announcements were made during intermissions, and Enough Is Enough T-shirts were thrown to the audience between periods of play.

The committee's focus during the remaining months of 2011–2012 was to widen the scope and help other constituencies on campus recognize when events fit within the Enough Is Enough initiative. The hope was to have the logo included on advertisements for all programs that address issues of violence on campus. These collaborations included the campaign's support of Rachel's Challenge (named after Rachel Scott, the first victim murdered in the Columbine High School shooting). Rachel's Challenge is a nonprofit organization dedicated to changing the lives of many by sharing Rachel Scott's story and asking audiences to start a chain of kindness and compassion in an effort to prevent violence. Additionally, the Enough Is Enough video was updated in the spring 2014 semester, and a Facebook page was developed to further educate the SNHU community about the importance of treating others with respect.

In 2012–2013, the second SNHU video was launched and the campaign included a week that focused on issues related to violence and bullying. Programs included Black and White Day, which encouraged members of the community to wear black and white to support the initiative. Additionally, a "hands are not for hurting" campaign and "positive tweet" communication drive occurred. Messages were presented about how to intervene if students witnessed another student being bullied or abused, or if they were concerned about a particular student. Example strategies included contacting public safety officials to report the incident, making noise to distract the perpetrator of the violent event and then getting help, and—when safe—simply making a statement to the perpetrator that identifies the behavior as abusive.

SNHU's Enough Is Enough campaign is included in freshman orientation and continues to be reintroduced to the entire community through some new programming initiatives (e.g., diversity programming, Take Back the Night, hazing prevention programs). Bystander intervention training is included at the annual student leadership conference, where backpacks with the Enough Is Enough logo and the new campaign slogan "I've got your back" are provided to participants. At the beginning of the spring 2014 semester, a message was sent to faculty and staff reminding them about the campaign and offering ways they could join the efforts to reduce violence. The Enough Is Enough message reaches students at the annual Involvement Fair, the Big Money Bingo game, and the Random Acts of Kindness Week during February. Other programs included working with Generation Equality on a NOH8 campaign; creating a video of students telling their stories about bullying; participating in a full month of activities in March titled "31 Days to Change the World," which included another presentation of Rachel's Challenge; and participating in a Color Peace 5K run on the first day of the national Enough Is Enough Week.

In order to assess the effectiveness of the campaign, a biannual alcohol and other drug survey went out to the student body that included the questions, "Have you intervened when another student was being bullied or physically or sexually harassed?" and "Were you bullied or physically or sexually harassed by another student?" In 2011, 38.9% of students reported intervening, whereas in 2013, 71% of students reported taking the initiative to stop incidents of bullying. In 2011, 92.7% of SNHU students reported they had not bullied or physically or sexually harassed another student. In 2013, 95.4% of students reported they had not bullied or sexually harassed another student (New Hampshire Higher Education, 2011, 2013). This indicated a decrease in the number of students who may have participated in an incident of violence, as well as a significant increase in the percentage of students intervening to stop the violence from occurring in the first place. The hope is that the awareness campaign is educating students on how to intervene and help protect their fellow students, as well as how to be a part of a community of peace.

The campaign is currently seen by the SNHU community as a vital part of keeping the campus safe. Student groups, faculty, staff, and community continue to offer their service to the committee and inquire about how they can promote peace. This yearlong campaign has a presence on campus and supports the university's stance on prevention of violence.

Recommendations

The rising rates of violent tragedies on college campuses across the United States highlight the need for prevention and intervention. Small colleges, in particular, face the challenge of developing and implementing prevention plans while also facing declining levels of staffing and financial resources. In order to ensure that these smaller institutions are able to provide a safe community, we encourage a number of specific strategies.

Identify, Assess, and Quantify the Issue

There has been growing concern about guns and other weapons being on campus, and it is important to assess and understand the relevant data. Unfortunately, there has also been much conjecture about how pressing the issue actually is on college campuses. In order to further understand the issue and the campus's needs, assessments need to be conducted with students, faculty, and staff. This assessment initiative should look at how many individuals report having a gun on campus, how many individuals would bring a gun if they were permitted, and what thoughts and beliefs exist on campus related to whether weapons should be permitted.

Create a Gun Safety Philosophy on Campus

If guns are permitted on campus, institutions should require annual training to ensure individuals have been properly educated on gun use and require gun holders to maintain appropriate state permits. Additionally, campuses should consider gun protection and storage protocols for students, faculty, and staff.

Identify Sustained Campus Leadership

In order for an antiviolence program to be successful, it is important to have a campus leader or "champion" express and encourage support. Unaware or resistant individuals can often overcome indifference or opposition to a new idea with the appropriate encouragement and support. Rogers (2003) and Schon (1990) agreed that either a new idea finds a champion or it dies. It is neither required, nor often desired, that the champion be a powerful individual with a high office. In this instance, a senior leader may be inaccessible to individuals who are doing the planning and implementing the new decision (Rogers, 2003). Schroeder, Mable, and associates (1994) found that midlevel managers are the most effective champions for new ideas if they hold a key position and possess analytical and negotiating interpersonal skills. In Rogers's research, champions became brokers for the new idea, shaping it to fit within the organizational structure. In negotiation and brokering, Rogers (2003) found that "people skills may be more important than power" (p. 415). After identifying a campus champion(s), it is important to establish a standing committee of dedicated individuals from across the institution to establish systematic and intentional antiviolence interventions, programs, and services. This committee must include members from across the academy and local community.

Create and Implement a Behavioral Intervention Team

One of the concerns raised during the investigations of the tragedy at Virginia Tech was the lack of communication within the university related to students of concern (Urbina, 2007). The recommendation that developed out of the investigations was for colleges and universities to develop behavioral intervention teams. It is important for small institutions to implement such teams, consisting of representatives from various departments within the college or university (see chapter 6 for more detailed information).

Maintain a Strong Counseling/Psychological Services Office

In recent years, higher education has seen more students with varying levels of mental health challenges and needs successfully attending college. Despite these increases, many small colleges' counseling office budgets have had no commensurate increase—and may even have decreased—while struggling to keep up with the additional work-load. To be clear, research has shown that those with mental health issues are more likely to be the victims of a violent incident than to be the cause. Nonetheless, in order to keep students safe, small institutions need to ensure that counseling and psychological services are adequately staffed, funded, and maintained (Kingkade, 2014).

Expand Violence Prevention Education

In an effort to follow and understand the current trends in violence prevention, small colleges and universities should expand their violence prevention efforts by joining campaigns, such as NASPA's Enough Is Enough program. By joining this or similar initiatives, member institutions will receive resources, tools, and suggestions on how to offer systematic and comprehensive programs and services to address this important issue.

In the end, gun violence and methods to prevent it are issues that colleges and universities will continue to face. Clearly, this is not a problem facing higher education alone, but one that will continue to challenge society until we address its underlying causes. Until that happens, small institutions have several tools that can help prevent incidents of gun violence. These tools, coupled with strong leadership and community commitment, may make a difference in keeping campus communities safe.

References

Birnbaum, R. (2013, September–October). Ready, fire, aim: The college campus gun fight. *Change: The Magazine of Higher Learning*. Retrieved from http://www.changemag.org/Archives/Back%20Issues/2013/September-October%202013/gun-fight-full.html

Drysdale, D., Modzeleski, D., & Simons, A. (2010, April). *Campus attacks: Targeted violence affecting institutions of higher education*. Retrieved from _http://www2.ed.gov/admins/lead/safety/campus-attacks.pdf

English, B. (2013, November 8). Some parents overly involved in college students' lives. *Boston Globe*. Retrieved from http://www.boston.com/news/local/massachusetts/2013/11/09/parents-overly-involved-college-students-lives/gqzLTGE6HI516O117VrMNJ/story.html

Kiley, K. (2012, April 19). Welcome to the party. *Inside Higher Ed*. Retrieved from http://www.insidehighered.com/news/2012/04/19/less-elite-colleges-well-versed-confronting-problems-think-they-can-teach-elites-few#sthash.WiDGNeVG.dpbs

Kingkade, T. (2014, October 7). Using college mental health services can lead to students getting removed from campus. *Huffington Post*. Retrieved from http://www.huffingtonpost.com/2014/10/07/college-mental-health-services_n_5900632.html

Luzer, D. (2013, July 26). The most important change coming to college: Fewer students. *Washington Monthly*. Retrieved from http://www.washingtonmonthly.com/college_guide/blog/the_most_important_change_comi.php

Marklein, M. B. (2013, October 23). Colleges see a slowdown in tuition price increases. *USA Today*. Retrieved from http://www.usatoday.com/story/news/nation/2013/10/23/college-tuitions-rising-more-slowly/3151897

New Hampshire Higher Education Alcohol and Other Drug Committee (NHHEAOD). (2011). NHHEAOD Resources. Retrieved from http://www.nhheaod.org/resources.htm

New Hampshire Higher Education Alcohol and Other Drug Committee (NHHEAOD). (2013, March). *Education Services–Enough is Enough*. Retrieved from https://my.snhu.edu/Offices/WellnessCenter/Pages/EducationalServices.aspx

Richman, J., & Emmons, M. (2014, January 16). Stockton shooting: 25 years later, city can't forget its worst day. *San Jose Mercury News*. Retrieved from http://www.mercurynews.com/ci_24928327/stockton-shooting-25-years-later-city-cant-forget

Rogers, E. M. (2003). *Diffusion of innovations*. New York, NY: Free Press.

Schon, D. (1990). *Educating the reflective practitioner: Toward a new design for teaching and learning in the professions*. San Francisco, CA: Jossey-Bass.

Schroeder, C. C., Mable, P., & associates. (1994). *Realizing the educational potential of residence halls*. San Francisco, CA: Jossey-Bass.

Selingo, J.J. (2013, April 17). Colleges struggling to stay afloat. *New York Times*. Retrieved from http://www.nytimes.com/2013/04/14/education/edlife/many-colleges-and-universities-face-financial-problems.html?pagewanted=all&_r=0

Urbina, I. (2007, August 30). Virginia Tech criticized for actions in shooting. *New York Times*. Retrieved from http://www.nytimes.com/2007/08/30/us/30school.html?pagewanted=all

U.S. Department of Education. (2014). *Campus crime statistics online*. Retrieved from http://www2.ed.gov/admins/lead/safety/campus.html

U.S. Department of Education, Office of Safe and Drug-Free Schools. (2010). *Action guide for emergency management at institutions of higher education*. Retrieved from http://rems.ed.gov/docs/REMS_ActionGuide.pdf

9

A Community Colleg
Perspective

Preparing for Active Shooter Events

Lance Jones and Scott Peska

"YOU NEED to get back to campus. We've had a homicide." These are words no one wants to hear, but they are what coauthor of this chapter Lance Jones, director of security at Casper College in Wyoming, heard when he answered his cell phone a few minutes after 9:00 a.m. on November 30, 2012. Having served in campus law enforcement for most of his life, he was no stranger to "Hey, Chief, guess what?" calls at all hours. This, however, was a first. The investigation revealed that on November 30, 2012, the estranged son of a faculty member at Casper College, a public 2-year college, entered his father's computer science course and shot his father with a bow and arrow. He then fatally stabbed his father in the chest and, after murdering his father, used the knife to end his own life. It was later reported that earlier at his father's home, the son had stabbed his father's live-in girlfriend, who was a Casper College mathematics instructor.

Unfortunately, community colleges are no strangers to violent attacks or gun violence and have the same likelihood as other institutions of being victimized by active shooter events. An online search, using a variety of search terms to find active shooter events at community colleges, returned reports of 14 fatal shootings since 2009. Like all institutions, 2-year colleges must be prepared for all types of attacks, from individually targeted active shooter events to mass shooting scenarios. Drawing from characteristics that set community colleges apart from their 4-year counterparts, this chapter explores the prevention, preparation, and response efforts of 2-year colleges regarding active shooter scenarios or violent attacks. Following the model of Zdziarski's (2006) crisis management process, this apter identifies potential threats and risks as an opportunity to mitigate or prevent crises from occurring. Before reviewing common prevention initiatives, preparation protocols, or response plans, first we must review the unique characteristics of community colleges and the students who attend them.

Community College Characteristics

The first step in analyzing threats or opportunities is to gain perspective on the type of students who attend community colleges and the institutional characteristics that set community colleges apart from other institutions. Community colleges and public 2-year colleges are most widely known for their open access mission and provision of multiple educational opportunities (e.g., developmental education, occupational education, baccalaureate preparation, community education) to a diverse student body (Cohen & Brawer, 2003). Two-year institutions may be large, multicampus, multidistrict colleges or small, single-building campuses. Community colleges are often as diverse as their student populations, yet despite their differences, there are numerous similarities that set them apart from other institutional types.

Three overarching commonalities reported by the American Association of Community Colleges (AACC) (2014) are location (e.g., commitment to open access and serving local industry training needs), variety (e.g., serving high populations of part-time students, first-generation students, developmentally underprepared students, older students, and minorities), and flexibility in course and program offerings. Another commonly known difference is that community colleges cost significantly less than their 4-year counterparts. The College Board (Baum & Ma, 2014) identified the average tuition and fees at a public 2-year college (in district) as $3,241 for 2013–2014 whereas the average tuition and fees during the same time frame at a public 4-year campus (in state) was $8,895. The funding difference is important; 2-year campuses are often limited in the type or intensity of resources, services, and programming that can be offered when compared to those provided at 4-year campuses. Also with less funding, community colleges likely have fewer full-time faculty and staff and a greater reliance on part-time staff and adjunct faculty, and community college administrators are known to wear multiple hats. These institutional characteristics shape how 2-year colleges plan and prepare responses to protect their diverse student body from violent active shooter events.

For the last 15 years, it has become common knowledge that, of all institution types, community colleges serve nearly half of all undergraduate college students in higher education and the largest percentage of first-generation college students. According to the American Association of Community Colleges (AACC), 2-year colleges in 2012 served 45% of all U.S. college students and 36% of 2-year college students who identify as the first generation in their family to attend college (AACC, 2014). Aside from the number of first-generation students, community colleges also serve the highest percentage of Hispanic/Latino students (56%) and Black students (48%) in higher education (AACC, 2014). Other common characteristics of community college students reported by the AACC (2014) are that the majority attend part-time (60%) and that they are non-traditional or older students (71% over the age of 21). With many community college students having additional responsibilities, such as part-time or full-time jobs, or caring for dependents, there are often periods of nonattendance, frequently called "stopping out." According to a recent study of 38,000 community college students in Texas, 76% of those who earned a bachelor's degree stopped out at least once and 94% of all community college students experienced a period of nonattendance (Vendituoli, 2013). Cohen and Brawer (2003) contended that community colleges are often the doorway to social mobility for low-income, minority, and underprivileged students. Diverse students bring a host of unique challenges and opportunities to community colleges that can both support and hinder their collegiate experience.

So what, if any, is the relationship between background characteristics and active shooter events? Aside from sex (e.g., most active shooters have been male), there are relatively few demographic variables that serve as good predictors of who might be involved in an active shooting. Research conducted by the FBI has shown that there is no accurate "profile" of students who engage in targeted school violence (Blair, Martaindale, & Nichols, 2014; Vossekuil, Fein, Reddy, Borum, & Modzeleski, 2004). Unfortunately, one background characteristic that is commonly linked with recent violent attacks on schools is mental illness, such as depression, anxiety, or post-traumatic stress disorder (PTSD). Many individuals with these conditions have demonstrated difficulty coping with loss or personal failure, and many have presented with suicidal ideation (Vossekuil et al., 2004). According to Grasgreen (2012), colleges and universities have seen an increasing trend of students with psychological needs. This may be a particular issue for community colleges because, unlike their 4-year counterparts, they often lack the resources (e.g., staffing) to adequately serve those with psychological needs. A study conducted by the American College Counseling Association's Community College Task Force, which surveyed respondents from 294 colleges in 44 states, indicated that 97% of community college counselors have additional responsibilities (e.g., advising, career counseling) beyond clinical counseling (Edwards, 2011). Although this can be viewed as a barrier to providing students with adequate mental health assistance, it also means trained counseling staff are connecting with students for other purposes, such as selecting their courses. This study also reported that 88% of responding community colleges indicated that they did not offer psychiatric services on campus or have a contract with a local provider (Edwards, 2011).

According to Gallagher (2013), who reported similar findings from a national survey of counseling center directors, 2-year institutions had nearly double the ratio of counselors to students (1:2,972) when compared to 4-year institutions (1:1,604). The same researcher reported that none of the community colleges in the study offered on-site psychiatric services and only 6% had on-site medical services, in comparison with 56% of the 4-year institutions offering psychiatric services and 67% providing on-site medical services.

These studies support the notion that community colleges lack staffing and resources to provide invaluable services that not only help their students but also provide the college an opportunity to better assess potential risks. Most community colleges (87%) reported not offering after-hours emergency counseling services, and just over half (53%) limited the number of counseling sessions students could attend at their institutions (Grasgreen, 2011).

Immediately after the bow-shooting incident at Casper College, the on-campus counseling staff responded to the location where students and staff were directly impacted by the incident. They were then sent to different locations to help those individuals who witnessed or were otherwise directly affected by the situation. Due to the need, numerous counselors from other entities in the city volunteered their services, which were coordinated by Casper College's Counseling Center director. Volunteers worked late into the night and throughout the weekend for any community member who wanted to talk. They also performed a yeoman service for the entire campus community.

Prevention Efforts

There is no evidence to suggest community colleges are more or less susceptible than 4-year colleges to experiencing mass shootings based on their institutional characteristics or the background characteristics of their students. However, these characteristics may make 2-year institutions susceptible to some vulnerability in their violence prevention and response planning efforts, which are different from other campuses. For example, after the shooting of Congresswoman Gabrielle Giffords, news reporters questioned Pima County Community College's failure to adequately warn the community of the shooter's dangerous potential (Grasgreen, 2011) because he was a former student with known "red flag" issues. It is extremely difficult for 2-year campuses to adequately track or monitor the communication and behaviors of their students because students largely commute to campus, attend part-time, and start and stop out frequently. Furthermore, counseling staff juggle multiple responsibilities. Traditional 4-year campuses have been perceived as having advantages, such as first-line residence halls staffed to assist in monitoring community members' behaviors, that community colleges lack (Grasgreen, 2011; Jaschik, 2013). Although residence halls bring their own unique challenges to a campus, the additional staff and increased opportunity to notice "red flags" are clear benefits. Additionally, there are often college apartments for rent near traditional, 4-year institutions, which provide a sense of closeness within the community and may also provide other students the opportunity to notice and report potential concerns. Relatively few community colleges offer residence halls. Edwards (2011) reported that only 20% ($n = 60$) of respondents to the Community College Counseling Services survey indicated having residential halls. According to Cohen

(2001), community colleges were often cautioned by states to not provide residence halls because their primary purpose was to serve students within the local community.

Since many community colleges do not have residence life staff, they rely on other frontline staff and faculty to identify threats and report concerns. However, prior research (Edwards, 2011; Gallagher, 2013) indicates that 2-year campuses generally cannot provide the same provision of student services, such as mental health counseling, as 4-year campuses. This is of concern because of the number of students attending all higher education who attend college with mental illness and depression. In 2007, the *Orange County Register* reported that 25% of students in the University of California system were taking antidepressants or related drugs and that about 10% of students had seriously considered suicide (Sforza). Whereas many 4-year campuses have support to help these students, some community colleges may not. Grasgreen (2012) suggested that all too often community college professionals have to wear many different hats, such as mental health counselors also serving as academic advisers or career service professionals. The Lone Star Community College system received criticism from the American Federation of Teachers (AFT) after a stabbing incident occurred on one of its satellite campuses in April 2013, just a few months after a shooting incident on a different Lone Star campus left three students dead (Jaschik, 2013). According to a report filed by the AFT, only three counselors were working on the campus, which serves approximately 18,000, when the stabbings occurred, and when the campus opened in 2003 it had seven counselors, who served nearly 6,000 students (Jaschik, 2013). The president of the AFT stated, "An important component of school safety is not just common sense gun control measures, but sufficient mental health services" (Jaschik, 2013, para. 14).

Many community colleges have an intervention and assessment team in place. The primary purpose of these teams is to provide a way for faculty, staff, and students at colleges to report suspicious student behaviors or communicate a potential threat. According to Cornell (2010), *threat assessment* can be broadly defined as identifying dangerous situations, whereas a narrow definition shared by the Federal Bureau of Investigation (FBI) and Secret Service centers on investigating an individual or group who communicated a threat or engaged in threatening behavior. Essentially, the purpose of these teams is to help determine if a threat has a likelihood of actually posing danger. In an article by Jaschik (2013) published in *Inside Higher Ed*, Daniel Carter suggested that community colleges face different issues in assessing threats than 4-year campuses. He argued that the open access mission, combined with many 2-year institutions having numerous campuses and often relying on local security and police to address and respond to violent attacks, can leave community colleges vulnerable (Jaschik, 2013). For example, in 2013 a shooting occurred at the New River Community College satellite campus located within the New River Valley Mall. The shooter wounded two individuals before he was apprehended by an off-duty mall security guard, as the college relies on the mall security company at that location. Although the local police arrived in five minutes and no one was killed, this situation could have been much worse. The 18-year-old shooter was reportedly returning to his vehicle when apprehended, and he complied with the unarmed, off-duty security guard (Griffin, 2013). The shooter reportedly posted information encouraging individuals to follow the public scanner for the New River Valley Mall just prior to entering and firing at people. Although prevention might not have been possible, community colleges with smaller satellite campuses often rely on local authorities or a shared security detail, which presents unique risks.

One risk that potentially faces some community colleges is a lack of adequate resources to monitor student behaviors and communications, which are critical to identifying and assessing potential threats (Vossekuil et al., 2004). As in the shooter case at New River Community College, many school shooters have revealed (before their attack) some threatening statements or behavior that prompted concern in others (Vossekuil et al., 2004). At Louisiana Technical College in 2008, a 23-year-old woman killed two other female students and herself. Reports indicated she had been living in her car and displayed signs of paranoia. She also alerted a crisis center to inform them that she planned to kill herself (Cornell, 2010). Another example, the 2009 shootings at Henry Ford Community College, involved a 20-year-old student who killed a classmate and himself after the instructor covered the history of mental illness. The shooter had posted YouTube videos expressing his hatred toward Black women and also shared his intentions to kill himself (Cornell, 2010). Des Moines Area Community College (DMACC) was able to detect a threat before it occurred through monitoring Twitter. The tweet called for volunteers to attack the DMACC Ankeny Campus while another shooter attacked the Urban Campus. The perceived threat was deemed noncredible by an assessment team, but due to the stringent zero-tolerance policy related to violence, the student was arrested on the second day of class ("Threat," 2011).

Threat assessment teams are essential at community colleges to bolster prevention efforts. With the high number of adjunct faculty members who teach at community colleges, there is a strong need for systematic documentation and communication about student issues and concerns. According to the Community College Counselors Survey (2013–2014) (American College Counseling Association, 2014), 88% of counselors who responded reported that their campus had a threat assessment team, or equivalent. This number has increased since the 2009–2010 survey (American College Counseling Association, 2010), which reported that 75% of institutions had these teams. Cornell (2010) suggests there are three critical features for threat assessment teams to be successful: administrative support, campuswide education and information about the threat assessment team, and cross-disciplinary team membership. Threat assessment teams should be an important part of any 2-year campus's violence prevention efforts.

Laura Bennett, president-elect of the Association for Student Conduct Administration (ASCA) and a community college conduct officer and campus threat assessment team coordinator, said this about the effectiveness of crisis action team/behavioral management teams at community colleges:

> An effective campus behavioral intervention team [BIT] or threat assessment team plays the critical role of a "safety net" for 2-year institutions. Through a multi-disciplinary lens, we evaluate behaviors to determine a level of risk, and employ appropriate interventions to prevent escalation toward violence. Without a resident adviser check on a student, a First Year Experience class, or a mandatory orientation to evaluate initial behavioral baselines, a well-trained community college BIT is a campus's best resource for preventing violence without over- or under-reacting, and violating students' rights. As Peter Langman states in his 2009 book *Why Kids Kill: Inside the Minds of School Shooters*, "The best defense is early detection. Shooters have to be stopped before they can get to the school with weapons. This means a different style of prevention than physical security." While I know not every act of violence can be prevented, threat assessment teams focus on early identifica-

tion and intervention to minimize the risk of violence and promote student success. In today's society, I can't imagine working at an institution without a threat assessment team. They provide faculty, staff, and administration a supportive place where any member of the campus can report unusual or concerning behaviors that might otherwise keep them up worrying. (personal communication, July 1, 2014)

In addition to identifying threats, community colleges need to understand how their students perceive safety on campus and safe areas on campus. Campus climate surveys can provide individual campus information regarding perceptions, perceived concerns, and awareness of safety or emergency preparedness resources. Recently, Patton and Gregory (2014) investigated perceptions of safety among students attending all Virginia community colleges and found that students attending a campus with no security or police force had the greatest concern for their safety. Moreover, there was a significant difference by age and enrollment status; specifically full-time, 18- to 24-year-old students felt safer than part-time, nontraditional students, likely because younger students take classes during the day, whereas nontraditional students take more evening classes (Patton & Gregory, 2014). Parking lots were among the areas on campus where students had the most concern for their safety at 2-year campuses (Patton & Gregory, 2014). Because many community colleges are commuter campuses, this finding was unsurprising. At Hazard County Community and Technical College, a 2013 parking lot shooting of three people left two dead. The suspect turned himself in to Kentucky State Police. He reportedly knew his victims, sharing a child with one, and the community college parking lot was simply the meeting location for exchanging their child for visitations (Kingkade, 2014). Community colleges should ensure parking lots are well lit, are patrolled routinely by security, and are equipped with safety measures such as emergency blue light call boxes. Additionally, community colleges should encourage students to be mindful of their surroundings and provide safety education strategies (e.g., walking in pairs) in their orientation and new student informational materials. However, due to limited staffing and resources at 2-year campuses, these safety recommendations may not be easily implemented.

In addition to lacking resident advisers, residential staff, or other first reporters, the programmatic offerings or individuals assigned to prevention duties by departments of public safety vary greatly between 2-year and 4-year campuses. According to Reaves (2008), 2-year campuses (62%) had fewer personnel designated for crime prevention compared to 4-year counterparts (94%) and fewer designated officers for various prevention and specific response duties (see Table 9.1). Further, students are not as available as on 4-year campuses. Thus, orientations at 2-year institutions may not be mandatory, and opportunities such as floor meetings that can bring in officers to speak to students are lost. Therefore, the issue of educating and training students in prevention and the available response services is a crucial one for community colleges.

Community colleges may have vulnerabilities associated with the characteristics of the institution (e.g., open access, heavy reliance on adjunct faculty, fewer resources) or with the students who attend community colleges (e.g., part-time attenders, commuters, adult students), which discourages the college faculty and staff from getting to know their students well. These same characteristics can, however, also be viewed as advantageous in planning, preparation, and response. For example, part-time, commuter, and older students

Table 9.1   Percentage of Institutions With Programs or Designated Personnel for Prevention and Response Services

	2-Year Campuses (%)	4-Year Campuses (%)
Crime prevention	62.0	94.0
Rape prevention	48.0	84.0
Self-defense training	48.0	84.0
Victim assistance	47.0	73.0
Stalking	42.0	77.0
Community policing	40.0	80.0
Student security patrol	39.0	66.0
Drug education	36.0	87.0
Cybercrime	35.0	75.0
Alcohol education	30.0	84.0
Bias/hate crime	28.0	64.0

Note. Adapted from "Bureau Campus Law Enforcement 2004–05," NCJ 219374, by B. Reaves, 2008, www.bjs.gov/index.cfm?ty=pbdetail&iid=411, p. 19.

may rely less on the institution for direct support in the aftermath of a tragedy as they have families, friends, and community resources nearby that they can turn to for help and assistance.

Preparation Efforts

There are many factors that come into play with respect to the preparation to respond to these violent crises. Staffing, assessment of and following an emergency response plan, training and annual exercises, relationships with community resources (e.g., police, fire, hospitals), and the role of campus security are just a few. It takes an annual assessment of campus emergency procedures, resources, and key personnel to ensure that campuses are prepared for the unthinkable. After the shootings at Virginia Tech and at Northern Illinois University (NIU), many campuses reevaluated their preparations based on the lessons learned from these shootings. Sometimes only after an incident can a campus truly learn where it needs to improve its preparation. Blair et al. (2014) suggested that civilians should also be trained on how to react, because they found that it takes approximately three minutes for police to arrive on the scene of an active shooting. The actions that faculty, staff, and students take to protect themselves are of critical importance. There are a variety of no-cost resources available to help colleges and universities, such as the video "Run. Hide. Fight" which is endorsed by the FBI, Department of Homeland Security, and Federal Emergency Management Agency (FEMA) (Blair et al., 2014). These types of trainings for faculty, staff, and students are geared to help individuals protect themselves and others until a police response arrives.

For instance, North Virginia Community College (NVCC) in 2009 experienced an active shooter who fired at an instructor. When his gun jammed, students fled and the assailant gave up, sat, and waited to be arrested. Tom Jackman (2010) with the *Washington Post* reported that a 16-page internal after-action review of the situation revealed that there were significant concerns regarding NVCC's preparation. Specific concerns were that campus police did not have access to floor plans or master keys to certain areas, that only 9 of the 45 security cameras were operational, and that the campus was not prepared to issue an immediate alert. Since then, NVCC has addressed these concerns and added additional security measures, such as installing lockable doors in all classrooms and alert PA systems at two of its satellite campuses (Jackman, 2010). Campuses must have systems in place to check their preparations and to ensure equipment, such as blue light call boxes or security cameras, are operational.

One of the factors for consideration in preparing a response is the decision to have armed or unarmed security forces. A recent study conducted by the Center for Naval Analysis reported that 42% of institutions interviewed ($n = 66$) did not have armed officers on campus in 2004–2005, but have since decided to arm their officers largely due to mass shootings (King, 2013). This is not an uncommon phenomenon. Although this study was focused mostly at 4-year universities, many community colleges have had or are having discussions to determine whether to arm their protection professionals. According to a study by the Bureau of Justice Statistics based on 2004–2005 survey data of 2-year and 4-year institutions with more than 10,000 students (Reaves, 2008), the average number of sworn personnel at 2-year campuses ($n = 14$) was less than half of the number of sworn police officers at 4-year campuses ($n = 32$). Although Reaves (2008) did not offer the ideal ratio per student, he reported that 67% of 2-year campuses had sworn police forces versus 96% of 4-year public campuses.

After tragic shootings, which gain national attention, many campuses report making or planning to make changes to their emergency management protocol or security/police force (Hattersley Gray, 2014). In 2007, the president of the California College and University Police Chiefs Association stated that approximately 60% of California community college security forces were armed (Sforza, 2007). An Internet search, using various search terms, such as *community colleges arming security* and *community colleges arming police* revealed news-related articles that indicated that since the Virginia Tech shootings in 2007, 10 community colleges have armed or were in the process of deciding to arm their security/police officers (Table 9.2).

The decision to arm law enforcement sometimes rests with the college administration or with the board of trustees. Mount Wachusett Community College's board of trustees recently voted to allow the college's police force to carry firearms on campus, beginning January

Table 9.2   Two-Year Colleges That Have Armed or Are Considering
Arming Their Campus Security or Police Force

College	Year Implemented
MiraCosta College	2006
Pasadena City College	2007
Estrella Mountain Community College	**2008**
Jackson State Community College	2011
Bristol Community College	2013
Carroll Community College	2013
Cleveland State Community College	2013
Holyoke Community College	2013
Greenfield Community College	2014
Mount Wachusett Community College	2014

1, 2016 (Hartwell, 2014). The president was initially opposed to arming campus police; however, he reversed his decision due to concerns over recent mass shootings (Hartwell, 2014). Another example is Cleveland State Community College, which switched from unarmed campus security to campus police due to violence across the country on school campuses (Cleveland Daily Banner, 2013). Wake Technical Community College, a five-campus network in North Carolina with more than 64,000 students, recently decided to create a police department following the heightened violent mass shootings and two separate gun-related threats of violence, which resulted in campus lockdowns in the same academic year (Jahner, 2012).

However, not all campuses can make the determination to arm their security forces at the campus level. In Connecticut, Manchester Community College (MCC) had to request approval from the Connecticut Board of Regents to arm its police force. All of the state's public 4-year campuses had armed police forces, but as of 2013, 10 of the 12 community colleges were not armed. In March 2013 at MCC, unarmed police received notice that a student had a gun in his waistband; they could assist local police only with logistical planning, despite having more knowledge of the campus layout and the ability to respond faster (Besthoff, 2013). Faster response times and better knowledge of campus layout are two important factors that community colleges must take into consideration when determining whether to arm their police force.

Shortly after the shootings at NIU in 2008, Waubonsee Community College, located approximately 25 miles west of NIU, made the decision to shift from security officers to an armed police force. Although the decision was made for a number of reasons, Waubonsee followed the lead of other Illinois community colleges that also made the transition to armed police forces (e.g., College of DuPage, Elgin Community College, Harper College, and College of Lake County). John Wu, executive director for emergency management and safety stated,

> Waubonsee's overall strategy to improve safety was to focus on prevention and preparedness. To that end, arming and training of officers serves only to improve our preparedness and response capabilities, but does little to further prevention efforts. Having an armed police presence on campus may deter some individuals considering mass shootings, but there's no way to know if that's enough. With Waubonsee's main campus situated in a rural setting we also wanted to increase our timely response and not depend upon city police who may have competing priorities. Having a recognized police department and actively participating in threat assessment teams offers opportunities to check criminal backgrounds, communicate quickly with area police agencies, remove threatening individuals from campus and serve warrants. The authority to take these prevention actions is what's really important. (personal communication, July 8, 2014)

A news story by the Associated Press indicated that McHenry County College discovered cost-saving benefits after the decision to switch from an armed security force to a police unit. The security force of 22 part-time and full-time employees was trimmed to 10 full-time sworn officers, and the budget dropped from $598,909 in 2009–2010 to $512,565 in 2013–2014 (Associated Press, 2014).

Despite some of these benefits, arming a campus police force may not always be the best option. Wolf (2014) reported that some of the risks of arming campus police forces include unjust or improper use of force, accidental weapons discharge, escalation of weapon use, and collateral damage to bystanders. Wolf (2014) also acknowledged that the downside of unarmed security includes putting the security guards, faculty, and students in possible danger. Community colleges that do not choose to employ their own police or security officers are reliant upon law enforcement services from the jurisdiction in which they are located. These jurisdictions could include police departments within the city, the county sheriff's department, or the state police, if the campus is located in an unincorporated area.

Following the 2012 attack, Casper College reviewed events and determined arming the security department would not have altered the outcome of the situation, and it remains unarmed today. A motion by some faculty members to be allowed to carry weapons on campus was not ratified by the faculty senate. Some other campuses have opted to forego campus security personnel altogether. Western Nebraska Community College (WNCC) has remained without security or armed officers. However, WNCC actively informs students how to respond to unlikely events during their new student orientation, has strengthened its mass notification alert to include local hospital staff, and routinely practices realistic drills with local law enforcement so off-campus officers know the layouts of campus buildings ("How UC Davis," 2011).

It is natural to focus preparation efforts on the immediate response to an active shooter event; however, campuses should also consider preparing plans to initiate recovery efforts should such an event unfold. Again, fostering relationships with key community partners is paramount in building recovery efforts. For example, having relationships with counseling agencies could be instrumental in providing enough resources at the time they are most needed by students. In the unfortunate event of death resulting from a mass shooting or active shooter response, campuses may be expected to host communitywide events, such as memorials, candlelight vigils, and so on. Having identified campus teams or individuals to lead certain projects could help reduce stress during the aftermath of an event and set the stage for positive, holistic recovery efforts for the community.

Preparation is essential for campuses, and decisions about whether to arm security teams or how to conduct training for faculty, staff, and students are issues community colleges must consider. In the unlikely event of an active shooter scenario, the campuses' and individuals' response efforts depend upon how well prepared they are. Preparation is the key to helping individuals make the best decisions possible when lives may be at stake.

Response Efforts

Relationships with local authorities are critical in order for community colleges to respond effectively in a crisis, as well as make recovery efforts after a crisis. Regardless of whether a campus has an armed police force or unarmed security, when tragedy strikes, a campus's support from community police agencies is invaluable to ensuring that a swift, comprehensive plan is well executed. In order for a college to build strong partnerships with external police (city, state, etc.) it must be forward thinking and make efforts to meet on a regular basis with external police to promote both campus and community safety. If that relationship is not strong, it may be perceived as ineffective or lacking thorough preparation. A strong partnership to consider is the "school resource officer" model employed in K–12 systems. The officer remains under the jurisdictional and operational control of the department through which they are sworn and assists the college on a day-to-day basis with campus safety and conduct matters. There are particular conflicts with this model, such as when the college may not want a particular situation handled in accordance with the general orders under which the officer must operate. For example, an officer may need to shift from a position of assistance to one of enforcement in relation to a faculty or staff member who has violated the law, and the campus community may find the arrest or use of force inconsistent with their sensibilities. Another conflict may arise if the officer attempts to become involved in behavioral conduct issues that the college prefers to address only via its conduct policy. Furthermore, a disconnect can occur if the officer is devoting too much of his or her time patrolling off campus, running traffic on the perimeter, or socializing with other police officers rather than being on campus.

If the college does not enjoy a good relationship with the city/county governments, or outside law enforcement simply lacks resources or professionalism, reliance upon outside law enforcement may not be a good model. Community colleges must have established trust in routine interactions so local officers responding to a crisis will not exacerbate problems.

At Casper College, police officers and agents from local, county, state, and federal agencies descended upon the campus in a unified response that demonstrated both speed and efficiency. The college security officers were included in the response efforts and played a supportive role for the police in providing keys and information as needed. Casper College security members were trained on the incident command system, and the preexisting relationships with police and fire departments enhanced the unified response effort. For example, prior to the incident, police and fire departments were provided with floor plans of every building and the chief of police, at the time, required city police officers to walk through all the school buildings within the city, including Casper College. The college security team hosted regular exercises on campus for first responders and met regularly with local emergency management officials. These actions led to a swift and decisive response to the violent bow attack in 2012.

Aside from differences between armed and unarmed protection or the strength of the town/gown relationship, community colleges may have slight advantages in several key areas of response. Generally, 2-year campuses have fewer buildings to protect than many 4-year campuses, so one advantage may be in the number of the facilities monitored. According to Reaves (2008) the number of campus buildings and the number of acres on campus were vastly different among institutional types. On average, 4-year campuses had 155 buildings and 878 acres, whereas 2-year campuses averaged 31 buildings and 240 acres (Reaves, 2008). Many community colleges use building sirens and loudspeakers to inform students of emergencies, which allows specific parts of campus to be effectively isolated. The emergency management communication plan about which mediums to use to deliver the message about the emergency may differ with each crisis. For example, a fire alarm may be activated to evacuate individuals; however, if there is an active shooter present, mass evacuation may not be the desired outcome. A loudspeaker announcement or alert-notification system may be a more appropriate and effective medium of communication.

A text-messaging notification alert system has become a popular method of informing campus community members of an emergency situation since the 2007 shootings at Virginia Tech. At Casper College, only a minute after the director of public relations was notified of the homicide, the school was placed on lockdown and the community was notified via text alert (Roerink, 2012). According to a *Campus Safety Magazine* mass notification survey (Hattersley Gray, 2014), campuses are investing in all types of security infrastructure, ranging from loudspeakers to text-messaging alert systems. Hattersley Gray (2014) compared the 2010 survey results to the 2014 survey results and found that text message notification system usage increased from 58% to 66% in 4 years. One challenge, however, with managing text message alerts is how the college enrolls students into the alert system. Some colleges, like Johnson County Community College, automatically enroll every student in the text alerts program and allow students to opt out on their text alert website. Montgomery Community College's text alert website allows students to opt in and encourages students to voluntarily enroll in this service (www .mc3.edu/about-us/text-alerts). In 2010, 15% of campuses were using social media for mass notification, compared to 38% using social media in 2014 (Hattersley Gray, 2014). In the 2010 survey, only 11% of campuses enrolled campus constituents via an opt-out model; the most common approach was to encourage new students to sign up through e-mail correspondence (47%) or new student orientation (47%). The 2014 survey results indicate that the opt-out option has gained traction, with 31% of campuses using this approach, a 20% increase, and that new student orientation (65%) was the most effective method of encouraging students to sign up (Hattersley Gray, 2014).

In addition to text alerts, many campuses communicate a "lock down" of their campus in an emergency as a quick response tactic. Whereas many 4-year campuses cannot truly "lock down" (e.g., prevent students entering or leaving campus grounds), achieving a true lockdown may be easier for some community colleges, due to the size and layout of the college. Although community college satellite campuses likely have less security coverage, or rely on local authorities for protection, they are often smaller and easier to "lock down." Often these campuses are single buildings or are located within an existing complex. Another security advantage that many 2-year colleges have is relatively few buildings on campus to protect. This makes it cost-effective for community colleges to have loudspeakers in each building or throughout campus as another local alert feature, compared to 4-year campuses.

An example of a 2-year institution that successfully used the lockdown procedure is Collin County Community College, in 2010, when a gunman lit a truck on fire outside to draw people out and then opened fire as they retreated (outside of the campus police station).

Reportedly more than 100 shell casings were found. The campus went on immediate lockdown, and within 3 hours the lockdown was lifted when the gunman was fatally shot during the exchange of fire (Hundley & Meyers, 2010).

Lessons Learned

Violence is not unknown among community colleges (Sforza, 2007). Community colleges that have faced active shooter events or mass shootings have the unfortunate opportunity to share what they learned from the experience—how they prepared and how they responded to the event. Every institution has a responsibility to maintain and restore the learning environment so that it is a place where students feel safe to continue to learn and develop without impediment or concern for their safety. Based on the community colleges' responses and empirical research done after mass shootings and active shooter events at 2-year institutions, there are a number of lessons that can enhance future response or prevention strategies at other colleges.

One of the first lessons is for colleges to be mindful of the connections and support offered by agencies, businesses, and municipalities in the communities that border them. In most of the examples provided in this chapter, it is clear that community colleges rely on the support of local law enforcement, often in greater capacities during a response than 4-year institutions.

For instance, at Casper College the partnerships at the local, state, and federal level were the cornerstone of Casper's ability to mitigate and respond quickly to a critical incident. Because Casper College lacks its own police department, it is vital that it maintains excellent rapport with first responders and emergency management officials within the community. One way this was accomplished was that Casper College security hosted the county's special response team twice for training with full-scale exercises, including active shooter scenarios. Community colleges should annually review protocols and building plans with local law enforcement agencies and practice facilitating systematic responses.

Another important lesson is to determine if the college's security team or police should be armed or unarmed. This decision is central to the role campus security or police will play in responding to these types of crises. As campuses reconsider or question arming their security or police force, it is important for community colleges to weigh the benefits versus the costs to their various constituents, one of which may be the relationship with current, local law enforcement and municipalities.

Another lesson is the notion of *lockdown*. Although this term may convey different meanings to emergency staff versus students or parents, it is imperative that community colleges determine what this means and educate faculty and staff about how to appropriately respond if enacted. Prior to the murders at Casper College in 2012, the majority of classrooms were only externally lockable. Afterward the campus invested resources to put new locks on the majority of classrooms and meeting rooms that allow for them to be locked from inside without a key. Additionally, while locks were being changed, faculty were issued wrenches to lock and unlock various doors from the inside.

Communication during emergency situations is critical. Casper College found that cell phone reception became unreliable after the shooting due to the high number of calls. Community colleges should talk to their cellular providers about increasing services during a crisis situation. Additionally, campus administrators should have backup communication plans ready. Casper College issued senior administrators and key personnel two-way radios in preparation for future emergency situations. Also, as previously noted, many 2-year colleges have begun utilizing text-messaging notification systems. Casper College also selected a new mass notification vendor, which allows students the opportunity to "opt out" of individual alerts while still remaining informed via a mass platform. In addition, the college reformatted its emergency response guide to make it more user friendly during critical events, and a new hard copy was issued to all Casper College faculty and staff and put online.

Another lesson learned is to take steps to prepare for the campus recovery efforts of a tragic event. Immediately after the imminent danger passed and the event was secured, Casper College had its food service vendor open to provide coffee and other refreshments at no charge to those impacted. Some students were waiting to be interviewed by police or had to wait because their cars were trapped inside the police perimeter, and this simple gesture provided a feeling that the college cared. Additionally, a few days after a tragedy, colleges may need to provide memorial services or similar events. At Casper College this included a candlelight vigil ceremony and an open mic–style gathering. These events bring community members together and provide a collective opportunity to grieve, which may greatly assist the healing process for many community members. Students and staff may create temporary memorials of items and messages, typically near the location of the shootings. At Casper, the classroom in which the violent attack took place was unused for nearly a year following the murder. It was thoroughly cleaned by a company specializing in such matters and remained closed until the community was ready for it to be reopened. Outside of this area became a temporary memorial until the classroom reopened; Casper placed a small, nonspecific plaque for the slain faculty members as a way to help the community honor the victims.

As Blair et al. (2014) suggested, colleges must help train citizens on how to respond within their settings. Since the attack Casper College has provided training, which included showing the employees the training video "Run. Hide. Fight." Casper also created a system of volunteer, trained "building marshals." In the event of a crisis, building marshals will ensure the building's exterior doors are locked, serve as a communication conduit between administration and emergency personnel, and assist in evacuation of the building as necessary. Additional training was provided for the campus security team, such as a train-the-trainer course in the ALICE (alert, lockdown, inform, counter, evacuate) Active Shooter Response Training system. The security team plans to offer training to building marshals and other campus community members as a means of preparation.

Another lesson from violent attacks since 2008 is the influential presence of social media. This includes information being gathered by campus officials from social media to inform the development of an incident or prevent violent crimes from occurring. The lesson also includes campus officials exploring how they may respond via social media after an incident occurs. This should be an important consideration community colleges address in the preparation phase. For example, Casper College's public relations department had to balance its desire to keep the community and other concerned individuals informed of developments in as close to real time as possible with police and fire departments requirements that all information released be properly vetted and presented as a single message from all agencies.

Although the lessons learned from previous active shooter or mass shooting attacks are invaluable, it is imperative to remember that no one model works for every campus. The important thing is to follow Zdziarski's (2006) process and assess the vulnerabilities, identify potential threats, and identify opportunities for improving methods of addressing violent attacks. Community colleges, like all institutions of higher education that have come under scrutiny, are often criticized or questioned for what they could have done to prevent or respond differently to such horrific crimes. According to Ferreia (1999), colleges must recognize their vulnerabilities; assess the probability and criticality of possible threats; and try to consider the motivation, potential, and capability of students who may commit such acts of violence. More than 85% of schools and universities indicate that they conduct a security risk/vulnerability assessment once a year or less (Hattersley Gray, 2014). Community college administrators need to be aware of the community resources and the importance that partnerships have in the response and continual assistance in the aftermath of a shooting. Faculty, staff, and administrators at community colleges should also be aware of the increased likelihood that a shooter is a local community member, compared to at a 4-year campus. Thus, sensitivity to the shooter's family and friends may be heightened at a 2-year institution, more so than among the students, faculty, and staff at a 4-year campus.

Conclusion

Although there is no single, silver bullet plan to slay the shape-shifting monster known as gun violence on college campuses, there are a number of strategies that community colleges can employ to minimize risk and strengthen response efforts. In summary, prevention efforts suggested for 2-year colleges in this chapter include, but are not limited to, the following:

> ➤ Conduct climate surveys about areas of safety/concern with
>   students.

➢ Inform faculty, staff, and students about identifiable risk/ threat factors.
➢ Use a threat assessment or behavioral intervention team to address concerning students or staff and to provide a clear, easy protocol for faculty, staff, and students to report their concerns.
➢ Provide prevention services and resources, despite having fewer personnel or resources; work with faculty; and package information in a format that can be received by the many different types of community college students.

In addition to prevention strategies, community colleges should focus on key aspects of preparation to address or redress violent attacks on their campus. The following are recommended preparation strategies:

➢ Establish ongoing relationships with local law enforcement and community agencies.
➢ Host trainings and practice response plans with local law enforcement to become familiar with the campus and emergency protocols.
➢ Train and educate all students, faculty, and staff using federally supported training resources.

Although responses will be different based on the unique characteristics of each 2-year institution and the context of the event at hand, the following response efforts should be taken into consideration:

➢ Maintain key relationships with community agencies and local law enforcement to ensure response efforts are coordinated.
➢ Use multiple communication channels for emergency purposes, such as loudspeakers, building systems, and text-alert messages, and train/educate students and employees during orientations.
➢ Create response and recovery plans with identifiable roles for individuals, such as building marshals, coordination of counseling services, and programmatic planning (e.g., vigils).

"Be prepared" is not a motto only Boy Scouts should live by; every institution should be as prepared as possible to address multiple emergency situations. According to a news bulletin released by the FBI, between 2000 and 2012 there were 110 accounts of active shooter events. Between 2000 and 2008, there were five active shooting events per year, rising to nearly 16 per year from 2009 to 2012 (Blair et al., 2014). This upward trend in active shooter violence means that everyday places, such as schools, churches, businesses, and colleges, must become prepared to address violent attacks. Through ongoing preparation and planning, when the unthinkable or unforeseeable occurs, your campus team will be ready to meet the challenge with efficiency, confidence, and a sense of readiness.

References

American Association of Community Colleges. (2014). *Fast facts from our fact sheet.* Retrieved from http://www.aacc.nche.edu/AboutCC/Pages/fastfactsfactsheet.aspx

American College Counseling Association. (2010, June 24). 2009–2010 *community college counselors survey results.* Retrieved from http://www.collegecounseling.org/community-college-survey-09-10

American College Counseling Association. (2014, August 29). *Community college counseling survey results.* Retrieved from http://www.collegecounseling.org/community-college-counseling-survey-results

Associated Press. (2014, July 3). Community college police boost security. *Community College Daily.* Retrieved from http://www.ccdaily.com/Pages/Campus-Issues/Community-college-police-boost-security.aspx

Baum, S., & Ma, J. (2014). *Trends in college pricing 2014.* Retrieved from https://secure-media.collegeboard.org/digitalServices/misc/trends/2014-trends-college-pricing-report-final.pdf

Besthoff, L. (2013, March 7). *Manchester police officer shot by fellow officer during college lockdown.* Retrieved from http://www.wfsb.com/story/21548726/manchester-police-officer-shot-by-fellow-officer-during-college-lockdown

Blair, J. P., Martaindale, M. H., & Nichols, T. (2014). Active shooter events from 2000 to 2012. *FBI Law Enforcement Bulletin.* Retrieved from http://leb.fbi.gov/2014/january/active-shooter-events-from-2000-to-2012

Cohen, A., & Brawer, F. (2003). *The American community college* (4th ed.). San Francisco, CA: Jossey-Bass.

Cohen, A. M. (2001). Governmental policies affecting community colleges: A historical perspective. In B. K. Townsend & S. B. Twombly (Eds.), *Community colleges: Policy in the future context* (pp. 2–41). Westport, CT: Ablex.

Cornell, D. (2010, January/February). Threat assessment in college settings. *Change: The Magazine of Higher Learning.* Retrieved from http://www.changemag.org/Archives/Back%20Issues/January-February%202010/

Edwards, J. (2011, Spring). *Survey of community/2-year college counseling services.* Retrieved from http://www.collegecounseling.org/docs/ACCA-CCTF-2011 SurveyBooklet.pdf

Ferreia, B. R. (1999). Risk management: A proactive program. In American Society for Industrial Security (Ed.), *Campus security and crime prevention* (pp. 5–12). Alexandria, VA: ASIS.

Gallagher, R. (2013). *National survey of college counseling centers: Section two: Comparison of 2-year and 4-year centers.* Retrieved from http://www.collegecounseling .org/wp-content/uploads/Survey-2013-2-4-year-center-comparison-2.pdf

Grasgreen, A. (2011, January 17). Could anyone have done more? *Inside Higher Ed.* Retrieved from http://www.insidehighered.com/news/2011/01/17/pima_ community_college_faced_challenges_with_loughner#ixzz33XZ6OGgF

Grasgreen, A. (2012, January 19). Too many hats? *Inside Higher Ed.* Retrieved from http://www.insidehighered.com/news/2012/01/19/community-college-counselors-face-challenges-survey-shows#ixzz33XZyhfRx

Griffin, J. (2013, April 18). *Off-duty security officer helps subdue Va. school shooter.* Retrieved from http://www.securityinfowatch.com/article/10924252/ alliedbartons-jim-gorman-subdues-suspected-school-shooter-at-va-mall

Hartwell, M. (2014, April 12). MWCC campus police gets OK to carry guns. *Sentinel & Enterprise.* Retrieved from http://www.sentinelandenterprise.com/news/ ci_25553136/mwcc-campus-police-get-ok-carry-guns

Hattersley Gray, R. (2014, May 5). Campuses continue to invest in emergency notification systems and upgrades. *Campus Safety Magazine.* Retrieved from http://www.campussafetymagazine.com/article/campuses_continue_to_invest_in _emergency_notification_systems_and_upgrades/notification

How UC Davis and WNCC prepare for campus shootings. (2011, May 2). *Campus Safety Magazine.* Retrieved from http://www.campussafetymagazine.com/article/ developing-an-effective-response-to-campus-shootings

Hundley, W., & Meyers, J. (2010, August 17). Gunman who opened fire on McKinney police department identified. *Dallas Morning News.* Retrieved from http:// www.dallasnews.com/news/community-news/mckinney/headlines/20100817-Gunman-who-opened-fire-on-McKinney-3579.ece

Jackman, T. (2010, June 22). Review: Virginia campus police responding to shooter did not have floor plans. *Washington Post.* Retrieved from http://www .washingtonpost.com/wp-dyn/content/article/2010/06/21/AR2010062104668 .html

Jahner, K. (2012, April 17). Wake Tech to add campus police force. *Campus Safety Magazine.* Retrieved from http://www.campussafetymagazine.com/article/college-plans-to-start-police-department

Jaschik, S. (2013, April 15). Threats at community colleges. *Inside Higher Ed.* Retrieved from http://www.insidehighered.com/news/2013/04/15/recent-incidents-point-challenges-community-colleges-facing-safety-issues#sthash .Wxx9pS3c.dpbs

King, D. R. (2013). Arming university police, part 1: The impact of mass shootings. *Campus Safety, 21*(7), 20–22. Retrieved from http://www.campussafetymagazine .com/article/Arming-University-Police-Part-1-The-Impact-of-Mass-Shootings/P3

Kingkade, T. (2014, January 13). There were more than two dozen reported shootings at college campuses in 2013. *Huffington Post*. Retrieved from http://www.huffingtonpost.com/2014/01/13/shootings-college-campuses-2013_n_4577404.html

Langman, P. (2010). *Why Kids Kill: Inside the Minds of School Shooters*. New York, NY: St. Martin's Press.

Patton, R. C., & Gregory, D. E. (2014). Perceptions of safety by on-campus location, rurality, and type of security/police force: The case of the community college. *Journal of College Student Development, 55*(5), 451–460.

Reaves, B. (2008, February). Campus law enforcement 2004–05. NCJ 219374. Retrieved from http://www.bjs.gov/index.cfm?ty=pbdetail&iid=411

Roerink, K. (2012, December 6). Casper College official, Casper police credit drills and alert system for quick response. *Casper Star-Tribune*. Retrieved from http://trib.com/news/local/casper/casper-college-official-casper-police-credit-drills-and-alert-system/article_a6b98991-2511-5883-b0db-ab077237b1ed.html

Sforza, T. (2007, April 26). Community colleges are not immune. *Orange County Register*. Retrieved from http://www.calstate.edu/pa/clips2007/april/26april/immune.shtml

Special to the Banner (September 11, 2013). CSCC transitions from security to campus police. *Cleveland Daily Banner*. Retrieved from http://nl.newsbank.com/nl-search/we/Archives?p_product=CDBB&p_theme=cdbb&p_action=search&p_maxdocs=200&s_dispstring=CSCC%20transitions%20AND%20date(all)&p_field_advanced-0=&p_text_advanced-0=(CSCC%20transitions)&xcal_numdocs=20&p_perpage=10&p_sort=YMD_date:D&xcal_useweights=no

Threat to shoot up Des Moines college campus draws quick response. (2011, August 30). *Des Moines Register*. Retrieved from http://blogs.desmoinesregister.com/dmr/index.php/2011/08/30/threat-to-shoot-up-des-moines-college-campus-draws-quick-response

Vendituoli, M. (2013, November 21). Are you a college stopout? New study says you might be. *USA Today*. Retrieved from http://www.usatoday.com/story/news/nation/2013/11/20/stopping-out-college/3647685

Vossekuil, B., Fein, R., Reddy, M., Borum, R., & Modzeleski, W. (2004, July). *The final report and findings of the safe school initiative: Implications for the prevention of school attacks in the United States*. Washington, DC: U.S. Department of Education, Office of Elementary and Secondary Education, Safe and Drug-Free Schools Program and U.S. Secret Service, National Threat Assessment Center.

Wolf, P. (2014, June). *F&M's decision to arm its campus police part of a nationwide trend*. Retrieved from http://lancasteronline.com/news/local/f-m-s-decision-to-arm-its-campus-police-part/article_d2f89f02-f8aa-11e3-990b-0017a43b2370.html?mode=jqm

Zdziarski, E. L. (2006). Crisis in the context of higher education. In K. S. Harper, B. G. Paterson, & E. L. Zdziarski (Eds.), *Crisis management: Responding from the heart* (pp. 3–24). Washington, DC: NASPA.

10 In His Words

The Tragic Reality

T. Ramon Stuart

LIKE MANY other students, when I enrolled at West Virginia University (WVU) in 1996, I anxiously anticipated the transition from high school to college. WVU provided the opportunity to pursue my educational dreams, although I also found myself fully engulfed in the many extracurricular activities available to students while studying at a university labeled as one of the top party schools in the nation. I must admit that I did everything in my power to help the university sustain this distinction.

For 3 years I served as a residential assistant in a residence hall that housed more than 400 residents, 50 of whom were on my floor. I initially assumed being a residential assistant as a creative way to finance college; however, I quickly realized the important role this position plays in the growth and development of college students. My experience as a residential assistant involved helping residents grow and develop into productive members of the university and society as a whole, despite the fact that many of the residents lacked the ability to visualize, articulate, and embrace their true purpose in life. The residents and I grew on a daily basis as we made monumental strides to expand our understanding of our university and our existence in the world. This helped many of us become better people as we existed within the imaginary protective gates of our university that shielded us from the dangers of the world.

My campus involvement expanded in 1999 when I pledged Alpha Phi Alpha Fraternity. My active participation at the chapter, district, regional, and national levels taught me how to interact with diverse individuals in an effort to find practical solutions to complex challenges. My fraternity experience and my work as a residential assistant allowed me to interact with a large cross section of students who elected me to represent them as a member of the 2000–2001 WVU Student Government Board of Governors (BOG) ("WVU Students," 2000).

My extensive growth and development in Alpha Phi Alpha, coupled with my ascension as a student leader, allowed me to hone my existing skills while developing a level of confidence that enhanced my critical thinking and decision-making abilities. This new skill set would prove beneficial during my college experience because it helped me develop an identity. I became comfortable with myself and my abilities. It also reinforced my sense of purpose because I realized my goal in life was to help others reach their potential. I did not realize at that time that developing my identity and defining my sense of purpose were essential to my psychosocial development while in college (Chickering & Reisser, 1993).

A former resident in my residence hall, Elizabeth "Beth" J. Sprague, died in her sleep on March 19, 2000, at age 21, from a condition known as cardiac arrhythmia (Kimm, 2003). Beth's unexpected death came as a surprise to those who knew her because she was athletic, energetic, and full of life. As a member of the BOG and because of my work as a residential assistant, I helped organize a memorial service for Beth so members of the WVU community could mourn her death. For the first time, many students who knew Beth faced the reality that death could strike at any time, even in the seemingly utopian world that existed on campus.

Beth's memorial service concluded with a bell-ringing ceremony conducted by the service fraternity Alpha Phi Omega. I felt at peace after the services because I was able to provide comfort to others during this trying time. Beth's death and my service to others required me to manage my emotions, which is an essential component of identity development in college students (Chickering & Reisser, 1993). The university community moved forward after our tribute to Beth, and I found myself doing the same by focusing on positive activities, such as enjoying friends and sporting events, and engaging in the classes necessary to complete my undergraduate degree.

My service as a member of the BOG concluded, and I completed my undergraduate degree in May 2001 prior to enrolling in graduate school at WVU the following August. Beth's death taught me and many other students at WVU that it was unrealistic to expect life to be perfect, despite the serene environment provided by our university. Beth's death triggered a transition in my life that further enhanced my growth and development as a college student. According to Schlossberg, Waters, and Goodman (1995), transition requires a situation that precipitates a change and the meaning that this situation has to the individual plays a critical role in how the individual copes with the transition. My ability to move through this transition in my life depended on how I personally viewed the event, the support I had, and the strategies I implemented to grow from the experience. At that time, I believed my development as a student and the transition caused in my life by Beth's death had prepared me to overcome any unfortunate situation.

Background

At approximately 7:30 p.m. on Saturday, February 2, 2002, my phone rang. The caller said in a calm voice, "Someone shot Jerry—come quick." The caller was referring to Jerry P. Wilkins. Jerry was a member of Alpha Phi Alpha and a sport management graduate student at WVU. I never imagined how my life would change that day as I raced to Jerry's apartment to evaluate the situation.

Paramedics were on the scene caring for Jerry as police officers placed yellow tape around the chaotic crime scene to prohibit bystanders from interfering. The situation appeared under control and certainly not life threatening, as Jerry sat in an upright position on the ground while paramedics tended to a single gunshot wound to his back. Within minutes, Jerry was in an ambulance headed to a hospital minutes away. Other students joined members of the fraternity and me at the hospital as the news of the shooting spread throughout the African American community. More than 50 students and several senior-level WVU administrators eventually gathered at the hospital, anxiously waiting for an update on Jerry's condition. Seconds turned into minutes, and minutes seemed to become days, as each of us wrestled with the events of the evening. We attempted to remain optimistic because we never imagined that a tragedy involving gun violence would occur on a campus like ours.

We shared memorable stories about Jerry to pass the time and to suppress our questions about his condition. Jerry was a proud man who knew what he wanted and was determined to acquire the finer things in life. He had recently completed an internship with a major record label, and he hoped to cultivate and hone his skills through an upcoming internship with a National Football League team. We laughed about Jerry's radiant smile and his charismatic personality that led his classmates to elect him as president of his graduate class. The stories of Jerry's antics and shenanigans produced joyful laughter in the waiting room; they provided comfort as we fought to ignore the reason we were gathered. These stories did little to prepare us for the reality of what was to come.

Due to my prior service as a BOG member, I knew many of the WVU administrators assembled at the hospital. One administrator called me to the emergency room. A sense of calmness fell over me as I walked into the room where there was little conversation before I heard the words, "He did not make it; Jerry is dead." Life seemed to pause; my ears heard the words, but my brain was unable to process the reality that Jerry died from a single gunshot wound. The calmness I experienced walking into the emergency room quickly turned to an acrimonious chill that pierced my body as my brain began to process the meaning of the devastating news.

One of the WVU administrators reached out to me to see if I felt comfortable announcing the news of Jerry's death to the students assembled in the waiting room that night. I agreed to deliver the news, believing my previous experience dealing with the premature death of my friend, Beth, prepared me for this task. I wondered what to say and how to say it, but I was unprepared to speak when the waiting room went silent as the administrators and I emerged from the emergency room. I informed everyone that Jerry died during surgery from the gunshot wound to the back. The room erupted with cries of sorrow and pain as the news resonated within each of us that Jerry was dead.

WVU provided a safe haven that shielded us from many of the horrors of the world, but that night we lost our sense of protection from evil when a murderer robbed us of our innocence by killing our friend and fraternity brother. Unwillingly, boys became men and girls became women that night in the waiting room of the hospital. Senseless gun violence on our campus caused the tragic death of our friend, and this tragedy left an indelible mark on our lives. Many of us struggled to prepare for the days ahead as our uncertainty forced us to operate in an unknown and uncomfortable environment as we sought answers in the aftermath of this tragic event.

Moving Forward

We left the hospital to go to Jerry's apartment, where we prepared for the arrival of his parents, who were traveling through the night to reach campus. We heard gospel music playing softly in the background as we walked through the door. The subtle rhythm and inspirational words provided a sense of peace; it appeared Jerry was in the right frame of mind prior to his murder. We struggled to find the appropriate words to say to Jerry's parents upon their arrival. Pain and anger were evident on their faces as they struggled to process the reality that their son was murdered while attending college. Our initial encounter with Jerry's parents made them realize the impact that he had on students at WVU, so they agreed to allow us to hold a memorial service on campus in his honor.

I organized and led the memorial service with the support of members of Alpha Phi Alpha and the WVU community. More than 600 people attended the memorial service, during which President David Hardesty remarked, "A great university knows its students one by one and, yes, we knew Jerry and we will miss him" ("Reward," 2002, para. 11), while Ken Gray, the vice president of student affairs, pledged unwavering support to aid students in the healing process. The memorial service concluded with a passionate appeal from Jerry's mother for information that would lead to the arrest of the person who killed her son. We boarded a university-sponsored bus days later to Philadelphia, Pennsylvania, where we laid Jerry to rest beside his grandmother, who passed away several weeks before.

WVU offered free counseling, and encouraged each of us to seek a peaceful resolution to this situation while avoiding the temptation to seek vengeance as we battled through the extensive and arduous healing process. Unfortunately, many students—especially members of Alpha Phi Alpha—failed to utilize the counseling services because we viewed doing so as a sign of weakness. Although unspoken, you could sense that members of the fraternity wanted to avoid the appearance of being vulnerable or cowardly in the wake of this tragedy. The emotions challenged our manhood—something each of us worked diligently to prove during our fraternity initiation process. The reality was that we were scared, and there was little anyone could do to change that. We were scared because someone killed Jerry, and we feared we, too, would become victims of senseless gun violence.

This fear prevented me from sleeping in my bed for more than a year after the incident. I believed I could confront any intruder who attempted to hurt me in my apartment because the assailant would expect me to be in the bed instead of the living room. I found myself being cautious about where I sat in public. I always positioned myself so I could watch the doorway for potential threats or make a quick exit. I remember one of my fraternity brothers sleeping with a large knife in case someone tried to attack him in his apartment. Many of us even contemplated purchasing a gun for protection, but I refrained because I was afraid of guns and the irreversible damage and pain that they can cause when used improperly.

We assumed the burial would be an opportunity for closure, but tears continued as we realized that an outstanding matter warranted our attention. It was time for us to relive the murder of Jerry as we prepared for the trial of the accused gunman—Brian B. Ferguson.

Trials and Tribulations

Brian was a fellow WVU student and most members of the fraternity knew of him from prior altercations with Jerry. One incident included several members of the fraternity physically attacking Brian at a party. That altercation, in addition to other relevant information received from students at WVU, led Morgantown police department detectives to investigate Brian's potential involvement in Jerry's murder. The investigation resulted in a first-degree murder indictment. To our surprise, Brian was released on bail after his arrest and arraignment until his trial began on November 19, 2002. This luxury afforded to Brian by our judicial system left many students at WVU, especially members of the fraternity, with a sense of fear and vulnerability.

I recall the night the WVU football team upset Virginia Tech 21–18. This triggered celebrations throughout Morgantown, including several couch burnings and excessive partying throughout the night (Kurz, 2002). Although he was on trial for first-degree murder, Brian visited a local nightclub to participate in the celebration. Those of us out celebrating that night left quickly because we feared retribution; it was public record that we were set to testify against Brian in his ongoing murder trial.

Although I played a minor role in the trial, the prosecuting attorney requested I testify about an incident Jerry shared with me. The incident involved Brian brandishing a knife and threatening to use it against Jerry if he continued a relationship of any type with Brian's girlfriend (*State v. Ferguson*, 2002). During cross-examination, the defense attorney asked several questions, and I answered each of them in a calm, matter-of-fact tone. However, I remember feeling like the defense attorney was trying to coerce me into saying things I had no knowledge of. The defense attorney eventually concluded the cross-examination after he realized my testimony was honest and did little to support his defensive strategy, which was to raise reasonable doubt that someone other than his client could be responsible for Jerry's death.

The judge allowed me to remain in the courtroom after my testimony, and I listened closely to the other witnesses. The testimony and cross-examination of each witness forced me to relive Jerry's murder in gruesome detail. The most difficult part was listening to the countless attempts by the defense attorney to depict members of Alpha Phi Alpha at WVU as ruthless gang members. These allegations were difficult to listen to as the defense attorney repeatedly attempted to vilify us—including Jerry. The defense attorney showed graphic autopsy photographs of the gunshot wound that killed Jerry, but he quickly drew the court's attention to the fraternity brand Jerry had on his body, suggesting the fraternity brutally branded members. He characterized this optional branding of Greek symbols as a member's commitment to protecting other members at any cost—even lying in court to convict an innocent man.

The defense attorney worked aggressively to discredit our words by going to great lengths to persuade the jury that we falsely accused his client because we were jealous of his wealthy upbringing. Brian took the stand to reinforce the claims of his attorney and to express his innocence. He appeared uncomfortable on the stand. He answered each question, but many of his answers seemed difficult to accept as logical and practical. Each answer seemed to be a well-crafted attempt to plant reasonable doubt in the minds of the jurors instead of proving he was innocent of killing Jerry.

On November 26, 2002, the jurors announced they had reached a verdict. We sat anxiously in the courtroom as the jurors emerged from the jury room to take their seats inside the courtroom. I remember listening to the verdict and expecting it to be a dramatic moment, like those depicted on television; however, the verdict came with little fanfare. Judge Robert B. Stone asked Brian to stand as the jury foreman read the verdict. Brian stood resolute as the foreman delivered a verdict of guilty of murder in the first degree with no recommendation of mercy.

Police officers placed Brian in handcuffs and led him out of the courtroom. We finally felt peace after months worrying about this tragic and unfortunate situation. There was no joy in the events that occurred, however. The gun violence essentially ended two young lives. We saw Brian again on February 24, 2003, as he entered the courtroom in an orange jumpsuit, handcuffs, and shackles. We listened as the judge sentenced Brian to life in prison without the possibility of parole (*State v. Ferguson*, 2002). Again, we were at peace; we no longer had to fear Jerry's killer. We never imagined that once the judge sentenced Brian to life without the possibility of parole that he would ever be a free man again.

Brian unsuccessfully appealed his conviction to the West Virginia Supreme Court in 2004 (*State v. Ferguson*, 2004). He then appealed to the U.S. Supreme Court in 2005 and was denied again. Brian filed a habeas corpus request in 2006, but the circuit court dismissed this petition the following year. He then appealed the dismissal of his habeas request to the West Virginia Supreme Court. That court ordered the circuit court to hold an omnibus hearing in 2011. The following year, the circuit court ruled Brian had ineffective counsel because another potential suspect allegedly confessed to Jerry's murder. The appellate court ruled that Brian's defense attorney failed to investigate this additional suspect thoroughly. The court granted Brian a new trial. The prosecutor appealed the ruling, but in October 2013, the West Virginia Supreme Court of Appeals affirmed the circuit court ruling to grant a new trial (*Ballard v. Ferguson*, 2013).

After serving more than a decade in prison, Brian is now a free man after the recent court ruling that granted him a new trial. The prosecuting attorney must decide if she will retry Brian for the murder of

Jerry, but this may prove to be a difficult task after all this time. The man once convicted of murdering Jerry may never serve another day in prison, and this reality produces many questions that are difficult to answer. Those of us who loved Jerry continue to live with the life sentence we received the night of his death, regardless of the current or future legal battles surrounding the murder.

Recommendations

As I reflect on the events of February 2, 2002, it is difficult to imagine the challenging decisions that WVU administrators had to make throughout this situation. No one expected gun violence to occur on our campus, but the university attempted to do all the correct things when it did occur. However, these efforts are ineffective and futile if students are reluctant or unable to accept them. As we are thrust into scenarios that require us to help students move forward and attempt to make sense of gun violence that occurs on campus, I offer the following recommendations based on my personal experience and knowledge of student identity theory.

Utilize Theory to Support Student Development and Transitions

The right thing to do in the wake of a tragic event involving guns is for administrators to pledge unwavering support to the campus community. This support is critical to the well-being of students, and it is essential to restoring order following a tragedy on campus. However, we should not wait until a tragic event occurs before we begin thinking about how to support the growth and development of our students. We must be proactive instead of reactive. Thus, it is imperative that we understand various aspects of student identity theory and the role theory plays in the growth and development of college students.

Chickering's theory of identity development offers seven vectors of development that help shape the identity of students (Evans, Forney, & Guido-DiBrito, 1998). Each vector plays a critical role in the developmental process of college students, and we, as academic administrators, must understand them if we want to effectively help students through difficult situations, such as an act of gun violence on campus. A deep understanding of how students develop while in college allows us to produce programs designed to foster this development. We can effectively design and implement programs throughout campus that engage students while helping them develop competence. This competence is an indicator to students that they can set and achieve goals. We can help students effectively manage their emotions by designing programs that teach students how to deal with a wide range of situations and individuals. We can support students' autonomy as we help them further develop confidence so they are able to create and maintain mature interpersonal relationships with various constituents on and off campus. Our ability to support this type of growth helps the student develop an identity that leads to a defined purpose in life. Lastly, our support of the growth of students allows them to develop a level of integrity that we hope students will adhere to in the classroom, around campus, and during interactions that extend beyond institutions of higher education.

Our application of student identity theory also provides us an opportunity to recognize student leaders while discovering students who may need additional support as they develop. This proactive approach prepares students for the unknown. For instance, I never imagined that my experience as a residential assistant and elected student official would prepare me for the tragic events that I faced while in college. These opportunities for growth provided me with the necessary tools that influenced my ability to deal with the death of a fellow student. Beth's unexpected death triggered a transition in my life that forced me to reconsider the roles I played in the world, my thoughts about life, and the types of relationships I developed and maintained with others.

Again, as administrators we must utilize our knowledge of theory to help support students during transitional periods. According to Schlossberg et al. (1995), transition involves situation, self, support, and strategies. We must help students make sense of tragic events that occur on campus as we help them understand how their background, beliefs, and various personal characteristics influence their view of the event. It is important that we provide appropriate support mechanisms to support students while they work to move through the ongoing transition caused by a tragic event on campus. Lastly, we must pause to consider the lessons we learn during a tragedy, and utilize these lessons to develop strategies that lessen the likelihood that future students will have difficulty transitioning after a tragedy.

The lessons I learned following Beth's unexpected death prepared me to deal with Jerry's tragic murder. This situation required me to rely on the leadership skills I learned as a residential assistant, through my involvement in the fraternity, and as an elected student leader while I sought the support of friends, family, and fraternity brothers to help me through the difficult transition.

We, as administrators, must look for more opportunities to encourage the growth of students because the experiences we create for our students position them to deal with a wide range of events, such as tragedies on campus and throughout life. Our understanding and application of theory allow us to help students as we prepare them for the realities of life.

Counseling Centers May Not Be for Everyone

I never utilized the counseling services offered by WVU following Beth's death or Jerry's murder, so I cannot argue for or against their potential benefits. What I can say is that many of the students I knew also failed to utilize the counseling services. The reality is that we did not know how to utilize the services offered. It was not that we did not know the location or the hours of operation of the counseling center. It was the fact that counseling was a taboo subject many of us would never discuss and a service we thought we would never utilize.

First, we were all struggling to cope with Jerry's murder. It was hard to imagine a counselor helping us through this difficult period because we had never interacted with a counselor before. Sharing raw emotions with a stranger was something I decided against because I fought so hard to prove I could handle the situation, and I wanted to stand strong in the face of adversity.

Second, members of the fraternity avoided counseling because we thought seeking help was an indication of our weakness and inability to manage this devastating situation like men. Fraternity members retreated to our sacred bond of brotherhood to provide our own support system. This was the only type of support we were comfortable with, and we relied on this informal support structure to get us through the tragedy. We turned to each other, but we always avoided the topic of Jerry's murder for fear of reliving the nightmare as we continued to struggle to make sense of the event that changed our lives.

We must find ways to meet students where they are and help them move forward in the wake of a tragic event on campus. Understanding that counseling centers are not for everyone is essential for academic administrators. In consideration of this reality we must find ways to expose students to counseling services available on campus before they are forced to consider using them. It is imperative that we develop messages that help us demystify counseling, and we must be diligent in educating students about the benefits of counseling after a tragedy occurs on our campuses. We must also find ways to enhance the support students receive through informal support mechanisms, such as fraternities and other groups students turn to, because, right or wrong, these entities are often more attractive to students looking for answers and support.

Empower Students to Act

The support of administrators at WVU empowered us to become change agents. Although this change was difficult to sustain once we transitioned from the university, it is refreshing to know that our work provided a foundation for future students to build on in an effort to eliminate gun violence at the university. Jerry's murder robbed us of a friend, but we gained a sense of accomplishment in the wake of the tragedy. For instance, after concluding Jerry's murder trial we looked for ways to remember Jerry and his contributions to WVU. We started initiatives aimed at increasing awareness of gun violence on campus with the support of WVU administrators. This was an opportunity for us to take steps to prevent future occurrences of gun violence at our university. We also used this tragic event as an opportunity to celebrate academic achievement by launching a scholarship in Jerry's honor that eventually became the Jerry P. Wilkins Scholarship for Leaders. This fitting tribute to Jerry's legacy provides financial support to a deserving minority student in the sport management graduate program at WVU who exemplifies extraordinary leadership skills while making great strides to improve the lives of others through selfless service ("Discounts," 2011).

Our institutions have many innovative and motivated students who feel great compassion following a tragedy on campus. We cannot stifle this compassion. Instead, administrators should find ways to motivate and cultivate student activism so students can bring about positive change. This active engagement is a productive use of students' time, and I personally found comfort in knowing my contributions played an instrumental role in creating something positive out of a negative situation.

Conclusion

I will never forget the events of February 2, 2002; family, friends, fraternity brothers, and fellow students at WVU lost so much that day. Yes, we lost a classmate, but we also lost our ability to shield ourselves from the evils of the world. We lost the ability to protect our innocence because someone used a gun to take the life of someone close to us. We were no longer immune to violence; instead, our exposure to violence forced us to develop a new sense of resiliency as we continued to develop as college students. Although the WVU community was supportive and nurturing during this trying time, many students, like myself, failed to understand the benefits of the vast resources offered by the university. We balked at these gestures of support as we struggled miserably to find ways to help ourselves. I am thankful WVU allowed me to grow on my own while I sought solace in familiarity and looked for ways to cope with this unimaginable situation. However, as an academic administrator, I argue that we can help students beyond just offering services we know many will not utilize to help them cope with a traumatic event that involves gun violence on campus. We can be proactive as we aggressively provide support to students before, during, and after a tragic event that involves guns on a college campus.

References

Ballard v. Ferguson, 12-1028 (The Supreme Court of Appeals of West Virginia October 25, 2013).

Chickering, A. W., & Reisser, L. (1993). *Education and identity* (2nd ed.). San Francisco, CA: Jossey-Bass.

Discounts for Greenbrier Classic alumni badges benefit Jerry Wilkins Scholarship Fund. (2011, May 3). *WVU Today*. Retrieved from http://wvutoday.wvu

.edu/n/2011/05/03/discounts-for-greenbrier-classic-alumni-badges-benefit-jerry-wilkins-scholarship-fund

Ferguson v. Ballard, 06-C-202 (2012).

Ferguson v. West Virginia, 546 U.S. 812, 126 S.Ct. 332 (2005) (denied Writ of Certiorari).

Evans, N. J., Forney, D. S., & Guido-DiBrito, F. (1998). *Student development in college: Theory, research, and practice.* San Francisco, CA: Jossey-Bass.

Kimm, M. (2003, November 5). *Sprague remembered.* Retrieved from http://www.connectionnewspapers.com/news/2003/nov/05/sprague-remembered

Kurz, H., Jr. (2002, November 21). All 'Eers: West Virginia picks off no. 13 Virginia Tech, 21–18. *Pittsburg Post-Gazette.* Retrieved from http://news.google.com/newspapers?nid=1129&dat=20021121&id=vvANAAAAIBAJ&sjid=u3ADAAAAIBAJ&pg=4963,122339

Reward offered in student's death; memorial fund established. (2002). *WVU Today.* Retrieved from http://wvutoday.wvu.edu/n/2002/02/27/1393

Schlossberg, N. K., Waters, E. B., & Goodman, J. (1995). *Counseling adults in transition* (2nd ed.). New York, NY: Springer.

State v. Ferguson, No. 02-F-95 (2002).

State v. Ferguson, 02-F-95 (2004).

State of West Virginia v. Ferguson, 607 S.E.2d 526 (WV 2004).

WVU students elect 2000–2001 student administration officials. (2000, February 25). *WVU Today.* Retrieved from http://wvutoday.wvu.edu/n/2000/2/25/3095

11

Violence Prevention in Modern Academia

Best Practices for Campus Administrators

Katrina A. Slone and Melanie V. Tucker

IN YEARS past, students entered college with the implicit expectation of safety within campus communities. However, following the devastating violence that has occurred at institutions of higher education in recent years, this assumption has greatly diminished. Regardless of whether a campus is small or large, private or public, community, technical, 2-year or 4-year, rural or urban, the previously held assumption that colleges are safe communities, a belief hitherto inherent within the fabric of their being, hardly seems accurate any longer. With violence increasing exponentially, it seems that safety within institutions of higher learning is decreasing exponentially to the point that constituencies may no longer expect safety, even within the classroom. Therefore, it is essential for administrators within modern academia to carefully examine proactive violence prevention initiatives.

Though administrators have grappled with campus safety concerns for years, the widespread and proliferating incidents of gun-related violence occurring on college and university campuses across the country have magnified and cast a glaring spotlight on this growing issue. One fact has become abundantly clear: "Recent tragedies demonstrate that campuses must be vigilant in identifying potential threats and develop coherent security strategies to effectively prepare for campus crises" (Harnisch, 2008, p. 6). The threat of gun violence, it appears, is not *if* it will happen, but *when*. To that end, it is essential for colleges and universities, regardless of size, location, or any other consideration, to implement strategies that will reduce the likelihood of violence. And, although little may be done to assuage the devastation of gun-related incidents that have already occurred on campuses across the country, there are best practices campus administrators may use to guide policy development and practical application in an effort to prevent the incidence of violence within higher education.

Best Practice 1: Develop a Comprehensive Weapons Policy

Critical to the core message of any university committed to reducing gun-related violence are the development and implementation of a clear, comprehensive, and, most important, effective weapons policy. The policy should address not only guns but also other weapons and the application of concealed carry within the state. Ideally, the policy works to achieve the highest degree of safety for the campus community while balancing the rights of gun owners. To achieve this, administrators must employ a multifaceted approach to policy development.

Consult Various Campus Groups

As policy development and information gathering processes begin, it is important for administrators to consult a broad range of concerned groups, both on and off campus. Faculty, staff, students, parents, alumni, and community members are in a position to contribute essential feedback within the policy development process. Additionally, it is important to consult key constituencies with a vested interest in policy implementation, such as campus security/public safety, law enforcement, risk managers, student conduct, residence life, and administrative teams designed to address threats, crises, and/or concerning behavior. These are the groups working on the front line and who will, predominantly, be the ones implementing and enforcing the university's weapons policy.

Clearly Define Terms

An important component to include within a weapons policy is a clear statement of the university's stance on concealed carry. Because a wide range of items may be considered weaponry, it is imperative that universities develop a specific definition of the term *weapon*. Although guns, knives, and explosives are consistently considered weapons, administrators must determine, for example, if equipment used within physical education classes, such as karate and self-defense, and equipment used by military-in-training groups are considered weapons. Moreover, allowances must be made for items that may inflict damage but are not traditionally perceived as dangerous accoutrements, such as baseball bats and other sporting equipment, kitchen knives, pocketknives, and toiletry razors. It is good practice to include a statement delineating how the possession of items that may appear to be weapons, such as toy guns, will be treated. Here, clarity is key; administrators must present an unambiguous definition that leaves no room for argument in the event of violations.

Provide for Exceptions

In encouraging administrators to be explicit about how *weapons* are defined, it should be noted that episodes of violence are rarely black and white. Therefore, weapons policies must clearly articulate repercussions for individuals who violate the policy, while allowing for some exceptions and flexibility. For example, select campus organizations (e.g., ROTC and other military groups, shooting and archery teams, martial arts) require weaponry as part of their functionality. Exceptions for these groups should be included within a weapons policy, while ensuring the campus community, including risk managers and administrators, is alerted to their presence and allowance.

The social and political climate of the region within the United States plays a major role in how the issue of guns on campus will be perceived. As a result, a practical appraisal should be undertaken of whether a complete prohibition of guns within the postsecondary sphere will drive some to conceal weapons, thus placing the task of risk management outside administrators' grasp. For instance, in areas where recreational activities such as hunting are popular, an excessively restrictive weapons policy will no doubt create much contention within the student, parent, and community populations, potentially engendering an atmosphere in which individuals feel compelled to illegally conceal weapons.

Provide Weapons Storage Guidelines

A weapons policy should also explicitly state how and where weapons should be stored. For example, some states allow individuals with concealed carry permits to store guns in their vehicles. Administrators should work with campus partners to identify areas where individuals carrying weapons may park, whether weapons are to be left in the vehicle or stored elsewhere, and, if stored elsewhere, how to transport the weapon to the storage location.

Publicize Policies

Once the weapons policy is fully developed, it is necessary to widely publicize it across the university community, including to students, faculty, staff, parents, and visitors. Guests at university functions, such as athletic events, art exhibits, lectures, and workshops, should have access to the policy and be aware that it also applies to campus visitors. An advertising campaign across various forms of media will help publicize the policy to groups on and off campus, as will integrating the policy into programming and training for students, faculty, and staff.

Additionally, administrators should consider how to provide access to the policy, whether in hard copy, through electronic media, or a combination of both (McCarthy, 2013; U.S. Department of Justice, 2005).

Evaluate and Revise

A detailed weapons policy is an essential component of every higher education institution's violence prevention strategy, and as with any plan, it is important to maintain an element of flexibility. Administrators should not be surprised if the policy evolves over time as changing legislation, political climate, and university conditions and needs necessitate (Scalora, Simons, & VanSlyke, 2010). Administrators should be prepared to make adjustments and keep in mind that policies addressing concealed carry and weapons are not one size fits all. Considerations must be made for the geographic location, campus size, number of buildings and venues, and population demographics as the intricacies of individualized policies are worked out (U.S. Department of Education, 2010). Lastly, what works well for one institution of higher education may not address the needs of another unique campus culture, and administrators must keep this in mind as they develop, implement, and publicize their weapons policies.

Best Practice 2: Implement an Emergency Operations Plan

A comprehensive weapons policy is one of many salient components of an emergency operations plan (EOP), which can help prepare the campus community to respond to gun-related violence, as well as other emergencies postsecondary institutions may face. The landscape of higher education in the United States, including geography, environment, institutional structure, and human capital, poses unique challenges for institutions when planning for and facing emergencies. Aspects such as consistently changing campus populations, access to high-level, security-laden research, and decentralized functions all contribute to increased vulnerability for campus communities (U.S. Department of Homeland Security, 2013) and need to be considered when administrators are developing and implementing their EOPs.

Gun-related campus tragedies at institutions of higher education have provided many "lessons learned" regarding the value of a fully informed and well-developed EOP, and the role of an EOP not only in campus safety but also in identifying protective and preventative measures for mitigating violent occurrences. The National Incident Management System (NIMS) (Federal Emergency Management Agency, 2014) provides a standardized foundation for developing postsecondary EOPs and serves as an excellent resource for higher education administrators seeking to implement an EOP. For institutions with an EOP already in place, reviewing the existing EOP within the scope of NIMS principles allows administrators to ensure their EOP meets or exceeds expectations and fits the current needs of the campus community.

Collaboration and Communication

Developing and instituting an EOP requires substantial collaboration and must include community and campus partners. Community partners, such as law enforcement, fire officials, emergency managers, public and mental health officials, and governmental representatives, can provide valuable resources and support in the midst of an emergency and play a pivotal role in communication (U.S. Department of Homeland Security, 2013). Campus partners, including but not limited to representatives from academic affairs, student affairs, facilities, administration, counseling and mental health, environmental health and safety, health services, human resources, information technology, legal counsel, public safety, housing and dining, disability services, transportation, and international student services, provide beneficial insight and information about the various constituencies on campus, contribute to the communication process, and play a role in educating the campus community. Collectively, strong partnerships on and off campus enhance administrators' ability to effectively navigate an emergency.

Communication is critical before, during, and after an emergency. As such, administrators would be negligent to not factor communication into their EOPs, as evidenced by the considerable media and societal attention paid to communication, or lack thereof, by institutions of higher education during recent campus tragedies (Eells & Rockland-Miller, 2010). Federal mandates, such as the Clery Act, the Family Educational Rights and Privacy Act (FERPA), and the Health Insurance Portability and Accountability Act (HIPAA), as well as antidiscrimination laws, such as the Americans with Disabilities Act (ADA) of 1990 and its amendments, Section 504 of the Rehabilitation Act of 1973, Titles IX and VI of the Civil Rights Act of 1964, and Title IX of the Education Amendments of 1972, play a role in information sharing through their varied mandates. Although administrators need to be aware of and proactive with decisions regarding emergency notification and timely warnings, they must also be knowledgeable about the applications and implications of mandates that dictate what may or may not be disclosed or communicated, when such information may be shared, and to whom.

Points to Ponder for Emergency Operations Plans

The ideal time for higher education administrators to consult with legal counsel regarding the institution's stance on communicating sensitive or protected information during a crisis and the potential for violating one or more federal mandates in the communication process is during the planning or review stage of an EOP's development, implementation, or revision. Informal discourse has illuminated that in light of public outcry in response to institutions not sharing information in the past, some administrators have decided they would rather go to court for disclosing too much information than not enough. This is just one example of challenging ethical decisions that may arise when implementing an EOP. Because higher education administrators must consider multiple perspectives and constituencies when developing their EOPs, difficult philosophical debates may ensue, about not only communicating but also matters pertaining to how to account for individuals on campuses that vary day to day; how to evacuate individuals with disabilities; or when to deny entry, lock down a facility, or shelter in place. Such questions may elicit emotional or reactionary responses from constituencies, and administrators must be prepared to help the campus community understand decisions before, during, and after an emergency.

The communication plans incorporated into an EOP are also critical when determining how to inform family members that loved ones are missing, injured, or deceased. Higher education administrators must follow law enforcement and medical examiner procedures for notifications; however, having trained personnel available to speak with and support family members in the short and long term is essential. Additionally, it is vital to have plans in place to provide support for campus community members. Thought should be given during the development of the EOP to considerations such as what will happen with facilities where gun-related violence occurs, the kind of support that will be given to faculty/staff who witnessed the violence, the kind of support that will be given to students, and whether there are functional areas equipped to provide support to some or all of the constituencies involved.

These are just a few of the many points for higher education administrators to ponder in order to develop and implement a fully informed, proactive, and actionable EOP. There are no easy answers, but administrators who take time to sufficiently plan and contemplate ramifications of different scenarios when not engaged in an emergency situation will be better prepared to lead their institutions during a crisis. By identifying what will work best for their individual campus communities and thoughtfully engaging in the process of developing and implementing an EOP, administrators may create a framework that will help enhance violence prevention initiatives.

Best Practice 3: Establish a Threat Assessment Team

Although the EOP informs senior administrators and the campus community during an emergency, campus constituencies may become aware of a threat prior to it developing into an emergency, and, if detected early, intervention prior to the threat escalating may be possible. As such, many institutions have established a threat assessment team, or an iteration of such a team, to assist with violence prevention efforts. Having this kind of team in place is quickly becoming standard within higher education, though one in five institutions still do not have one (Eells & Rockland-Miller, 2010).

A threat assessment team functions primarily to identify individuals who may pose a threat to the campus community and implement interventions designed to minimize threats once they are identified, before they become an emergency. Such teams serve a cross-campus function, communicating and collaborating regardless of silos; they exist to serve the best interest of the campus community. When functional, threat assessment teams prevent concerning behavior from "slipping through the cracks" and work to "connect the dots" between pieces of information across campus, creating a fully informed scenario upon which to act.

Factors such as campus culture and team membership substantially impact the functioning of threat assessment teams. Teams focused on the campus community with a commitment to building a campus culture of care will most successfully navigate challenges as they arise. Chapter 5 provides significant detail about threat assessment teams.

Best Practice 4: Create a Crisis Response Team

A crisis response team (CRT) serves the institution by responding to crises regardless of whether the EOP is enacted. Although the CRT should function as a part of the EOP, a fully developed, well-trained CRT allows administrators to implement an initial response to crises using limited human and financial resources. A student-focused CRT allows institutions to develop and implement a cross-functional team that can provide a broad and comprehensive response to student crises, as well as serve as a part of the prevention efforts on campus.

A student-focused CRT should be appointed, but not chaired, by the vice president for student affairs officer (VPSA) at the institution. As the VPSA will be serving in a leadership capacity in the midst of gun-related violence and other emergencies, the chair of the CRT should be the next in command, one level below the VPSA. This individual must be empowered to make decisions in the absence of the VPSA and capable of leadership in the midst of a crisis. Members of the CRT should include representatives from key functional areas, reflective of various student populations across campus, who have responsibility and authority to effectively address the needs of the campus community. Although each campus has unique characteristics that should be factored into the makeup of the CRT, at a minimum, the team should include the VPSA; the chair; the directors of counseling, housing, student activities, and student health; a public relations liaison; and key diversity officers (Hephner LaBanc, Krepel, Johnson, & Herrmann, 2010). Lastly, thought should be given to creating a backup system, secondary participants who would be called upon in the absence of a team member and should be included in team building and training activities as an effective redundancy plan.

Just like with the threat assessment teams, administrators should work with legal counsel to develop policies and procedures that inform the CRT work and are informed by federal and state mandates. CRT members should be trained on the policies and procedures specific to the CRT, as well as be knowledgeable about how the CRT aligns and functions with the EOP. Administrators should ensure that the CRT meets regularly and, further, encourage the CRT to hold tabletop exercises, both of which allow the CRT to develop as a team, increase efficacy, and identify educational opportunities for the campus community. Administrators should also support and encourage the CRT to maintain relationships with key constituencies on and off campus, including law enforcement, emergency personnel, hospitals, legal counsel, and community resource providers.

Victim Liaisons

An additional component that administrators should consider when developing a CRT is creating victim liaisons (Jablonski, McClellan,

& Zdziarski, 2008). Although victim liaisons do not typically serve on the CRT, they may be called upon to provide support for victims of a campus crisis. While CRT members should be appointed to the team based on their role on campus, victim liaisons should be selectively and specifically recruited based on individual characteristics that will best serve the institution during crises. Training for victim liaisons must be broad and include considerations such as the role of the liaison as an agent of the university; legal considerations; communication expectations, including privilege, privacy, and confidentiality; and resources and programs (Hephner LaBanc et al., 2010). Additionally, victim liaisons should be trained in "psychology first aid," as each crisis situation is unique, and liaisons must be prepared to respond to a myriad of emotional reactions.

A student-focused CRT provides another avenue for administrators to establish a feeling of safety, even during a crisis. When a CRT is able to quickly respond to and minimize the impact of a crisis, campuses are able to more quickly reestablish a sense of normalcy. By efficiently responding to student crises and assisting victims in transitioning back into the academic environment of the campus community, CRTs can positively contribute to administrators seeking to foster a sense of safety.

Best Practice 5: Implement Communications Systems

Whether implementing an emergency notification system campuswide or tweaking select aspects of an existing system, certain proactive, communication-based practices will ensure institutionwide success (Gray, 2012). Although no standardized, one-size-fits-all approach to campus communications exists, a multitude of options are available for consideration. The important factor to remember is that during a crisis, critical, lifesaving messages and information must be delivered and received with little room for error.

Emergency Notifications

Administrators should conduct an analysis of necessary communication components of the emergency notification plan, gauging the current level of functionality, and making sure to involve appropriate departments, like information technology, to determine feasibility. The plan should include the use of multiple technological sources (e.g., text and phone messages, e-mails, website updates, social media, tele- and videoconferences) to relay alerts, and include methods that are accessible for individuals with hearing and/or visual disabilities, as well for those who may not be able to receive "traditional" alerts. Certainly, emergency alerts need to be clear and concise; here, communication departments may provide leadership to ensure written and audible messages are direct and easily understandable.

Key individuals who have the authority to issue emergency alerts should be identified by administrators and receive proper training. Additionally, emergency systems need to be tested periodically. Administrators must alert the campus community members that emergency messages received during a defined time frame are only for testing purposes, but systems must be tested during busy, high-traffic times, as well as during slow usage times, to accurately gauge the notification system's effectiveness on a large scale. Marketing and education, both on and off campus, regarding the system are also important, ensuring individuals know how systems work during an emergency and also how to connect with the systems prior to an emergency (Gray, 2012). Like other emergency procedures, administrators should continue to make adjustments and alterations to plans as institution needs evolve.

Alternative Means of Communication

Emergency notification systems must utilize *multiple* alternate means of communication in emergency situations. During emergencies, traditional forms of communication (e.g., cell phones and landlines) quickly become overloaded, making information delivery impossible. Administrators should be prepared with accessible handheld radios and walkie-talkies, for example, and include communication methods that do not rely solely on power (e.g., battery operated). Increasingly, societal dependence on technology is detrimental in times of crisis; simpler methods may prove more effective. Administrators should not be nervous about devising approaches that fall outside the traditional realm of communicating. Institutions have reported using, to great effect, nontraditional forms of message delivery, such as fire alarms, hotlines, bullhorns, campus-runners who are assigned to deliver information on foot, and even police cars sharing information over loudspeakers (Schaffhauser, 2007). Naturally, the type of communication used is dependent upon the type of emergency involved. Therefore, the ability to extemporize appropriate modes of communication fitted to the situation is necessary.

Communicating With Various Groups

In relaying emergency notifications to constituents, both on and off campus, a fully operational mass communications system is absolutely critical. Information passed to those living and working on campus, local and state law enforcement, and families must be timely, and, most importantly, it must be accurate. However, administrators must be cognizant that the quantity and kind of information relayed to each group vary widely.

Communicating with the campus. Certainly, understanding the audience who receives emergency notifications will determine the type of messaging sent. For students, faculty, and staff, e-mail alerts, text messaging, and cell phone calls are arguably the best form of delivery—to a certain extent. Students and employees alike typically have easy, frequent access to both e-mail and text messages on their mobile devices, and these communication methods often prove effective in message distribution. Administrators must be mindful, though, that social media plays a major role in crisis alerts. Although an institution may not prefer or officially endorse social media for communicating emergency information, the proliferation of this kind of messaging is, indeed, extreme. For instance, during the Virginia Tech shooting in 2007, student-posted Facebook messages relayed and identified each and every victim a day in advance of traditional media's knowledge (Tinker & Vaughn, 2012).

Administrators should keep in mind that individuals possess the capability of spreading information, potentially erroneously, to parents and the outside community. This is when the importance of effectively managing the message becomes paramount. By managing the information the media receives, administrators cut the risk that fallacious and detrimental information might spread (Gray, 2012). With abundant access and availability of video, audio, and photographic capabilities on mobile devices during emergencies such as gun-related violence, higher education institutions encounter the danger of truly graphic images being leaked online. Administrators should be mindful that information not shared by the institution will almost certainly be shared for it.

Communicating with law enforcement. During an emergency, institutions must be able to communicate timely and accurate information that will save lives. A mass communication system that is interoperable with outside agencies aids in easy communication among campus police, local and state law enforcement officers, and first responders (Applied Risk Management, 2008). Interoperability of campus and local law enforcement officials means that essential players are able to reach out to each other "across disciplines and jurisdictions via radio communications systems, exchanging voice and data with one another on demand, in real-time, when needed and as authorized" (Major Cities Chiefs, 2009, p. 6). Because potential threats arise from a wide array of sources (e.g., threatening students and employees, participants in campuswide events), it is important that communication between agencies remains as smooth as possible (Major Cities Chiefs, 2009). Again, implementing multiple channels of communication delivery to outside responders is necessary; if one system breaks down, it is imperative to have others in place that will push the message through.

Communicating with parents and families. When relaying crisis information to students' parents and families, it is important to control the message during and after the event. Parents want to be able to quickly contact their children during an emergency; however, their influx of calls, texts, and frantic attempts to communicate may add unnecessary congestion to an already overloaded campus system. Therefore, administrators should identify factual, straightforward, and concise ways to proactively relay information to relatives (Greene & Greene, 2008). Provisions should be made to communicate with parents and family members of students who live in other countries, as well as with family members who do not speak English as their primary language. Establishing links with the institution's multicultural and foreign language departments and drafting preset messages will ease the communication process with families of students who speak languages other than English. Reassurances that all possible efforts to ensure and reestablish campus safety are in effect should be communicated in succinct and plain language. Administrators may also want to invest in the technology to house a call-in center through which additional call volume can be handled. Once the situation is resolved, appropriate messages should be sent to notify family.

Timely and accurate communication is paramount for administrative success during a crisis. Regardless of the constituencies requiring information, administrators must have multiple and varied ways in which to communicate— to not only minimize danger but also provide assurance that danger has passed. Implementing a thoughtful and thorough communication system is fraught with challenges and opportunities; yet it is an essential element of building the foundation for addressing campus violence.

Best Practice 6: Create Memorandums of Understanding

For smooth communication and implementation of emergency services, regardless of an institution of higher learning's size, location, or resources, it is important to establish links with agencies outside the campus community. Proactively establishing working relationships with key community partners, including local law enforcement, first responders, local medical services, emergency medical technicians, paramedics, and mental health providers, allows administrators to efficiently and effectively seek assistance in an emergency. For postsecondary institutions seeking to formalize agreements with off-campus entities a memorandum of understanding (MOU) is not only extremely beneficial but also often necessary.

Key Components of a Successful MOU

Any successful MOU contains several key components, including an introduction, overview of goals and purpose, a listing of agencies involved, along with the authority and jurisdiction of each, and a description about how and under which circumstances the MOU will be used. Successful MOUs clearly outline the responsibilities held by each agency, identify the chain of command, denote who is responsible for oversight, establish the duration of the MOU, and define the conditions under which the MOU may be modified or terminated. Finally, there should be a signature portion for the executive or lead official for each agency involved (U.S. Department of Homeland Security, n.d.). Administrators should have MOUs reviewed periodically to ensure relevancy, altering and enhancing as needed.

Law Enforcement Teams

Many campus law enforcement and security teams are simply not equipped to handle the multitude of demands expected of them during a large-scale disaster. When crises do occur, it is important to have MOUs with local and state law enforcement to alleviate some of the duties smaller or community colleges do not have the resources to manage (Applied Risk Management, 2008). Administrators should seek to create and develop strong partnerships with local law enforcement agencies prior to an on-campus incident. The implementation of a campus liaison officer to serve as point person between campus police and local law enforcement can greatly aid in opening lines of communication. In addition, regular meetings and training exercises will further facilitate smooth communication during crisis operations. A number of factors, such as technology, protocols, training procedures, and chain of command, which align with NIMS, must be navigated for an MOU to be successful. Although the coordination and development of interagency agreements can prove complex, the long-range benefits of developing MOUs far outweigh the challenges associated with instituting them (Major Cities Chiefs, 2009).

Local Health Agencies and Key Community Partners

In the interest of violence prevention and preemptive care, it is helpful to establish MOUs with local mental health agencies, primary care providers, and other health-related community partners. Whether provided on or off campus, mental health support and interventions substantially decrease the risk of violence and minimize danger campuswide (American Psychological Association, 2013). Furthermore, in the event of gun violence on campus, alliances with mental health organizations have proven critical in providing short- and long-term supplemental supportive care to those affected (U.S. Department of Education, 2007). The trauma and ongoing anguish suffered by individuals on campus who witness graphic violence and/or death may be significant, and the importance of having systems in place to provide assistance to these individuals cannot be overstated.

By creating MOUs with key partners, postsecondary institutions are able to form beneficial relationships and gain access to indispensable resources. The benefits of such alliances are multifold, allowing for provision of resources not only during crises but also when services may not be provided by higher learning institutions. Through thoughtful development of MOUs, administrators can make substantial progress in fostering caring communities on and off campus.

Best Practice 7: Foster Student Buy-In

In order to move a safety agenda forward in higher education, student buy-in is necessary. Unfortunately, although society has been shaken by gun-related campus tragedies, campus communities experience student-on-student-related violence on a regular basis. Such violence tends to occur in relatively public settings and often involves third-party participants or bystanders who are frequently students (Epstein, 2002). As such, fostering a campus culture in which students are willing to share information with and seek assistance for others could go a long way in reducing violence, particularly because students are more likely to persist at institutions in which they feel connected and are involved, both in and out of the classroom (Bogue, 2002). Cultivating student buy-in requires a multiprong approach, with careful consideration given to prevention education, collaboration with student organizations, clearly spelled-out student conduct codes and sanctions, and proactive identification of how to communicate with parents and families.

Prevention Education

Certainly, some people question whether violence prevention is possible in light of the limited ability to accurately predict violence. However, prevention education for reducing violence is focused on promoting healthy behaviors, providing assistance to those considered at-risk, and intervening with those who have demonstrated violent tendencies; it is not focused on predicting future behavior (Cornell & Guerra, 2013). Such an approach requires universal (primary) efforts focused broadly on the general student population, selective (secondary) efforts focused on students with increased likelihood for violence, and indicated (tertiary) efforts to mitigate future violent behavior in currently violent students. Administrators should seek to implement prevention efforts that are multifaceted, directed at multiple constituencies, and align with systems and structures already in place within the institution.

One area in which administrators may wish to focus prevention education is programming that addresses gender attitudes toward guns and gun policies. Although administrators must be cautious about gender stereotyping, women, in general, more often favor gun restriction and control policies than men (Mankowski, 2013). Therefore, prevention education programs aiming to alter perceived social norms among men regarding beliefs about masculinity stereotypes may effectively reduce interpersonal violence (American Psychological Association, 2013).

Another area in which administrators may seek to focus prevention education is bystander intervention. Bystanders with information about potentially violent or threatening situations often do not know what to do with the information or are afraid to come forward (Epstein, 2002). Bystander intervention education has developed in recent years following the proliferation of interpersonal violence. Evidence shows that students who have received bystander intervention education are more likely to intervene than students who have not been exposed to such education (Fischer et al., 2011).

Prevention education should also focus on psychological first aid (Scrivner, Tynan, & Cornell, 2013). Such training does not replace professional mental health services. It does, however, provide a way for students to help reduce the stigma associated with mental health treatment and puts additional skills into the hands of peers, who are likely to be the first to hear about threatening or concerning gun-related behavior. Targeting training to student opinion leaders, as well as key student groups, such as residential advisers, athletes, service organizations, and Greek letter organizations, can positively impact campuses' abilities to respond to crises.

Collaborations With Student Organizations

To foster and develop student buy-in, administrators should collaborate with student organizations. Doing so increases the viability of prevention initiatives. Collaboration may also reduce contention and protests arising between students who support concealed carry and those who do not, while also acknowledging basic rights, such as freedom of speech. Certainly, higher education administrators recognize the importance of the formative college years, during which some students explore new ideas, seek to find their voice, and strive to find their place in the world. By partnering with student organizations, administrators are in an ideal position to proactively prevent campus violence by working with student leaders to minimize conflict between those who oppose gun rights and those who advocate for such rights. This is of paramount importance for administrators at institutions who have experienced a gun-related tragedy and within communities who have experienced gun violence. Here, emotions about concealed carry may be heightened, and opinions may be particularly strong.

Administrators should also be aware of and knowledgeable about contemporary movements related to college students and violence. For example, some students have organized campus-based entities, such as Students for Concealed Carry (concealedcampus.org), to advocate for postsecondary students and employees to be allowed to bring guns on campus under concealed carry laws. In recent years, Students for Concealed Carry (n.d.) have begun hosting empty holster protests annually on campuses across the country to spark debates and send the message that gun-free zones create an attractive target for violent individuals. Additionally, nonstudent entities have created programs targeting college students, like the "NRA University," or NRA U (www.nraila.org/take-action/nra-university), provided by the National Rifle Association Institute for Legislative Action (NRA-ILA; 2014). NRA U is a 2-hour program designed to educate college students about the Second Amendment, gun safety, legislative threats, and ways to protect gun-related freedoms on and off campus. By staying up-to-date about these and other such organizations, administrators will be better equipped to stay ahead of these potentially undermining efforts. Administrators will more effectively seek and understand student concerns in order to shape the campus discussion while minimizing campus disruption.

Student Conduct Codes and Sanctions

It is the responsibility of campus administrators to ensure student codes of conduct clearly and succinctly express behavioral expectations. To that end, if the institution maintains a strict, no-violence-tolerance policy, that code should be communicated to students along with the sanctions associated with violations of the code. Conversely, administrators should consider including an honor code that speaks to bystanders sharing observations and concerns; it may offer some type of protection for students who report concerning behavior. Students may worry about retaliation and be hesitant to "snitch" on other students. Proactively putting measures in place through the student code and/or honor code will assure students it is in the best interest of all to report concerning behavior. Further, assuring students that privileged information they share will remain, as much as possible, confidential can help administrators cultivate student buy-in.

Sharing Information With Parents and Families

Just as behavioral expectations should be clearly communicated to students, they should also be clearly communicated to students' parents and families. Parents, guardians, and students should know what kinds of information will be shared when student conduct codes are violated. Parents and families should also be made aware of gun-related policies, gun-storing options on and off campus, campus student safety initiatives, and how to make referrals regarding concerning student behavior. Although it may seem counterintuitive to have parents or family members report concerning behavior, there are a variety of reasons why this may occur. For example, social media connects multiple generations, and it is not uncommon for parents or family members to discover concerning posts online. By educating families and parents about where and how to report such concerns, administrators take another step toward addressing safety while addressing concerns before they reach a crisis level.

Student buy-in, as a part of community building, is essential for moving a campus safety agenda forward. The more students feel connected to the campus community, the more they feel valued and included, and the more likely they are to persist. Administrators who are able to engage students in safety initiatives may more powerfully impact community building, both on and off campus.

Best Practice 8: Foster a Community of Care

Administrators seeking to foster a community of care must develop a shared vision of community, with common language and agreed-upon definitions implemented across campus, that provides purpose-driven goals for violence prevention efforts. As a comprehensive community approach for reducing violence recognizes that no single effort is sufficient, administrators should be mindful that there are a myriad of opportunities for effective prevention through programming, educating, and community building (Scrivner et al., 2013). Community-building efforts need to be aimed at all campus constituencies, with intentional efforts directed toward students, faculty, and staff.

Administrators in today's higher education encironment may experience challenges when attempting to balance the public demand for consumable education, which does not readily lend itself to community building, with the need for a caring community to collectively strive toward violence reduction and prevention. For administrators seeking to build a community of care, doing so must become an inherent component of the campus culture. This can be achieved by including community-building principles in activities such as strategic planning, marketing, professional development and training, leadership and service opportunities, and diversity initiatives (Moore & Carter, 2002).

One example of consistently implemented community building principles is demonstrated in the seminal report *Campus Life: In Search of Community*, in which Ernest Boyer (1990) wrote about how the community-building constructs of purposeful, open, just, disciplined, caring, and celebrative can foster and shape campus community. Boyer's community-building principles have been exemplified in efforts to build campus leadership, common experiences, and service opportunities; they have even been built into campus compacts, student pledges, and honor codes with the express purpose of engaging constituencies with community building. The salient aspect of community building is to develop a sense of caring about one another, of being invested in one another, which informs administrative functioning on a daily basis.

Reducing Stigma Regarding Mental Health Treatment

Key to creating a community of care is reducing the stigma attached to seeking and receiving mental health treatment. This has become a national agenda item, evidenced by the 2013 U.S. presidential plan for reducing gun violence, titled *Now Is the Time* (White House, 2013). Administrators seeking to reduce mental health stigma should work in tandem with prevention education initiatives across campus, including functional areas such as counseling centers, health services, student organizations, and academic departments. Efforts should be made to recognize that the inclusion of individuals with invisible disabilities, including mental illness, positively contributes to the diversity and richness of student life.

Achieving the goal of reducing stigma requires countering the misperception that only individuals with mental illness are responsible for gun-related violence. Although there is little link between mental illness and violence (Kadison & DiGeronimo, 2004; Peterson, Skeem, Kennealy, Bray, & Zvonkovic, 2014) and "individuals with serious mental illness commit only a small proportion of firearm-related homicides" (Cornell & Guerra, 2013, p. 3), assumptions continue to be made that violence is perpetrated by individuals who are mentally ill. It is important for administrators to help their campuses understand that most individuals who have a mental illness are not dangerous; but, for those students at risk for violence due to mental illness, mental health treatment can often prevent gun violence (American Psychological Association, 2013).

In creating a community of care, administrators should be aware that postsecondary students may come to college without an understanding of their mental health or the impact their mental health can have on their ability to be academically successful (Bertram, 2010), and that traditional-aged students are at a prime age when some major mental illnesses are first diagnosed. Students experiencing mental illness for the first time may choose to self-medicate or ignore concerning behavior and may not seek resources or support on their own. Some student populations, such as those who have been victims of personal violence, whether through war, natural disaster, gangs, shootings, or domestic abuse, may be quick to resort to violence or self-harming behaviors and may struggle to accept mental illness diagnoses, counseling, or psychotropic medication (Hollingsworth, Dunkle, & Douce, 2009; Parks, Wilson, & Harper, 2010). Campus communities that are able to respond to students with mental illness from a place of caring will be more effective in countering stigma.

Administrators should work with students and the campus community to identify ways to lessen shame affiliated with seeking assistance. That being said, administrators should also be aware of mandates that require mental health clinicians and medical professionals to report individuals who seek psychiatric hospitalization or individuals who are considered a threat to themselves or others. Although the need for mental health treatment should outweigh the concern of state reporting, such reports can disqualify individuals from becoming properly credentialed in their chosen career, such as law enforcement, law, or medicine, as well as being able to purchase a gun or be approved for a concealed carry permit.

The role campus communities play in reducing violence is still being explored, but it is clear that to achieve success, community efforts must be cross-functional and disregard silos that tend to exist on college campuses. Collaborative problem solving, joint initiatives, and intentional partnerships are all necessary to develop a sense of community and shared responsibility (Scrivner et al., 2013). Administrators who successfully develop a community of care may effectively prevent the disintegration of their campus's safety and embed intentional practices for increasing safety into the fabric of campus culture.

Best Practice 9: Educate the Campus Community

Campus policies and procedures aimed at violence prevention are most effective when members of the campus community are aware of and knowledgeable about them. Providing education to campus community members must occur in a variety of ways and be available ongoing. Additionally, consistent educational effort will cement the campus community's stance on gun violence and further develop a community of caring.

Safety Classes and Seminars

From the onset, each institution of higher education should develop and implement a series of educational safety classes or seminars accessible to all students, faculty, staff, and other affiliated parties. The U.S. Department of Education (2010) rec-ommended, as the most efficient and effective way to provide edu-cational information to the campus community, an "all-hazards" approach to safety classes. This method allows administrators to cover a broad range of potential emergencies, threats, and disas-ters, encompassing everything from natural disasters and severe weather to violence and terrorism, without requiring a separate course for each topic. Certainly, some threats will carry more weight than others. For example, emergency procedures for an active shooter on campus should be given more attention than campus actions during a power outage. There are a myriad of online training resources available to administrators (e.g., the Clery Center for Security on Campus) that provide a host of train-ing seminars, presentations, and videos, with both online compo-nents and in-person options.

Crime Prevention Programs

Imperative to the success of campus safety and security education is the development of plans for responding to violence as well as proac-tive programs designed to anticipate and assuage such episodes. This is where comprehensive crime prevention programs come into play. Through behavior intervention, threat assessment strategies, and crime prevention programs, institutions of higher education across the country have shown definite reductions in on-campus attacks (Deisinger, 2009). Use of Crime Prevention Through Environmen-tal Design (CPTED) allows administrators, law enforcement offic-ers, and planners to incorporate safety into the campus's physical environment through four principles: access control, surveillance, territorial reinforcement, and maintenance. When functionally employed, CPTED has been shown to "encourage a reduction in the fear of crime, a reduction in the actual number of crimes, an improvement in community safety, an improvement in the percep-tion of safety, and an improvement in the overall quality of life in a community" (National Crime Prevention Council, 2009, p. 1). The National Crime Prevention Council offers a multitude of training options specifically designed to assist campus administrators with understanding and implementing CPTED, as well as a host of other crime prevention strategies.

Security Awareness

As important as all-encompassing campus safety education initiatives are, promoting and developing security awareness can often prove challenging, particularly as law enforcement officers are sometimes viewed through an adversarial lens. At institutions that house public safety departments, it is crucial that all members of the campus community understand the importance and mission of such departments so they may fully cooperate with their security personnel (Scalora et al., 2010). Administrators should facilitate trainings and networking opportunities to create a greater sense of security awareness, including programming for employees and students to learn about safety policy and procedures (American Psychological Association, 2014). Fully functioning security measures require all aspects of campus life to work together toward a unified safety plan.

Educating Parents and Family Members

When it comes to a campus's safety and security, postsecondary ecosystems undoubtedly include a broad array of interested parties. However, one of the last groups to receive safety information and educational resources is often parents and families. Sharing information with parents and families can be a tricky issue because it typically involves students who have reached a legal age and, therefore, certain types of communication are legally limited (Greene & Greene, 2008). For that reason, administrators should ensure that parents and family members are aware of what kind of information is or is not typically shared and employ creative methods to ensure critical safety information can be disseminated.

Some institutions have dedicated a section of their institutional website specifically to parent information and programs. Administrators seeking to share information in this way should consider providing parent- and family-friendly sections, like "Frequently Asked Questions" with links to campus resources and "Vital Information" with essential security information and links to emergency services parents should know. Additionally, proactively sharing information about on-campus events like Parents' Weekends, Parents' Clubs, and Parents' Programs through parent- and family-specific e-mail communications, newsletters, and other publications, establishes strong ties linking parents to campus. These practices open lines of communication between parents and administrators in noncrisis-related ways and do much to allay fears experienced by parents of traditional-aged students.

How to Report Concerning or Threatening Behavior

Establishing detailed and comprehensive educational initiatives to ensure a safe campus is imperative, and essential information should be easily accessible at all times. The campus website should have a dedicated security section that lists resources, emergency numbers, and campus safety policies and information. All students, faculty, staff, and parents should be aware of how to report concerns to threat assessment teams and/or behavior intervention teams. This creates a mutually beneficial environment in which campus constituents feel comfortable confidentially reporting potential threats and voicing concerns and also provides a leg up to assessment teams as they work to address concerning behaviors early and correct problems in the collegiate atmosphere (Deisinger, 2009).

Best Practice 10: Conduct Campuswide Active Shooter Drills

Holding an active shooter drill provides a hands-on learning environment for campus administrators, law enforcement officers, students, faculty, and staff, and demonstrates the effectiveness of violence prevention policies and procedures with educational and community-building initiatives. Such drills serve as necessary diagnostic tools that allow the campus community to pinpoint areas within its emergency response plan that require additional enhancements and develop meaningful solutions to sharpen an institution's response to crisis situations through additional educational and/or community-building efforts. Although full active shooter drills may prove time-consuming and challenging, these types of exercises are critical to determine how the campus community and affiliated agencies will respond during actual crises.

Inform Constituencies

To avoid widespread panic and minimize unintended emotional or psychological impacts, administrators should consider conducting drills during off-peak times, such as between academic sessions or when human traffic is low on campus. Additionally, administrators should extensively publicize the time, date, location, and series of events that will occur as part of the active shooter drill through multiple communication channels. Messaging should occur in the weeks and days leading up to the event and reach constituencies on and off campus. Additionally, first responders, local law enforcement, and emergency medical personnel not involved in the drill need to be informed to curtail false alarms (Gilliland, 2014). The lasting impact of negative media, parent, and public response to a poorly executed active shooter drill can be detrimental and severe.

Inform the Media

Because of the widespread press surrounding gun violence on post-secondary campuses, it is important to be intentional about when and how to inform the media about routine emergency drills. It may be best to get ahead of the intense scrutiny that occurs, even during routine emergency drills. The campus's public information officer or media liaison should determine whether to disseminate information to the press, assuring them that the utmost precautions will be exercised, and safety of faculty, staff, students, and involved parties will be maintained (U.S. Department of Education, 2007). Media advisories, when sent, should include basic details like the expected time frame, location, and drill participants.

Debrief Afterward and Make Necessary Revisions

Following drill completion, administrators should debrief with all relevant participating parties. This allows important review of the events to determine which aspects of the drill worked well and which sections require improvement. Hindsight will shed new light on amendments that must be made and will allow administrators to adjust campuswide priorities to better protect lives. After adjustments and enhancements have been made to policies and procedures, additional educational or community-building initiatives should be identified to inform the campus community and continue to proactively address violence prevention. Holding active shooter drills that exemplify a high degree of emergency planning and preparation not only sets up institutions of higher education for success in the event of on-campus gun violence, but also promotes a culture of capability and resiliency among faculty, staff, students, and community partners.

Conclusion

Where once it was unfathomable to consider multiple gun-related tragedies at institutions of higher education, such events have unfortunately become frequent news headlines over the past decade. Violence prevention initiatives are always evolving, and although there is no one prescribed method that higher education administrators can follow to eliminate all interpersonal violence, there are established best practices that may move safety agendas forward and effectively reduce campus violence. Such practices can be categorized into initiatives surrounding policy and procedure development and initiatives related to educational and community building.

Within policy and procedure development, administrators should seek to develop a comprehensive weapons policy, implement an EOP, develop a threat assessment team and a student-centered CRT, institute multilevel communication plans, and create MOUs with community partners. Within educational and community-building initiatives, administrators should foster student buy-in; develop a community of care; implement educational programs for the campus community; and hold campuswide practice emergency exercises, including active shooter drills. Administrators must work with partners on and off campus to develop, implement, evaluate, test, and update policies, procedures, programs, and efforts aimed at violence prevention. Such efforts, though time-consuming and requiring buy-in from multiple constituencies, may result in reduction of campus and interpersonal violence, which is surely worth the effort.

Collectively, initiatives to prevent violence are intended to assist higher education administrators with creating campus communities in which scholarly activities and pursuit of knowledge can be supported. Campus administrators are encouraged to proactively engage in efforts to enhance campus safety, even though safety-related conversations are politically charged as fear abounds regarding rising rates of interpersonal violence. By taking a stand against violence and garnering administrative, campus, and student support for decreasing violence, administrators can foster safe campus communities that will effectively aid violence prevention.

References

American Psychological Association. (2013). *Gun violence: Prediction, prevention, and policy.* Retrieved from http://www.apa.org/pubs/info/reports/gun-violence-prevention.aspx

American Psychological Association. (2014). *Gun violence prevention.* Retrieved from http://www.apa.org/topics/violence/gun-violence-prevention.aspx

Applied Risk Management. (2008, June). *Campus violence prevention and response: Best practices for Massachusetts higher education.* Retrieved from http://www.mass.edu/library/reports/CampusViolencePreventionAndResponse.pdf

Bertram, M. (2010). Student mental health: Reframing the problem. *About Campus, 15*(4), 30–32. doi:10.1002/abc20033

Bogue, E. G. (2002). An agenda of common caring: The call for community in higher education. In W. McDonald & associates (Eds.), *Creating campus community: In search of Ernest Boyer's legacy* (pp. 1–20). San Francisco, CA: Jossey-Bass.

Boyer, E. L. (1990). *Campus life: In search of community.* Lawrenceville, NJ: Princeton University Press.

Cornell, D., & Guerra, N. G. (2013). Introduction. In American Psychological Association (Ed.), *Gun violence: Prediction, prevention, and policy* (pp. 3–6). Washington, DC: American Psychological Association.

Deisinger, G. (2009). *Developing and implementing campus-based threat assessment teams.* Retrieved from http://rems.ed.gov/docs/EMHETraining_SATX08_ThreatAssessmentTeams.pdf

Eells, G. T., & Rockland-Miller, H. S. (2010). Assessing and responding to disturbed and disturbing students: Understanding the role of administrative teams in institutions of higher education. *Journal of College Student Psychotherapy, 25*(1), 8–23. doi:10.1080/87568255.2011.532470

Epstein, J. (2002). Breaking the code of silence: Bystanders to campus violence and the law of college and university safety. *Stetson Law Review, 32*(1), 91–124.

Federal Emergency Management Agency. (2014). *National Incident Management System.* Retrieved from http://www.fema.gov/national-incident-management-system

Fischer, P., Krueger, J. I., Greitemeyer, T., Vogrincic, G., Kastenmuller, A., Frey, D., . . . Kainbacher, M. (2011). The bystander-effect: A meta-analytical review on bystander intervention in dangerous and non-dangerous emergencies. *Psychological Bulletin, 137*(4), 517–537.

Gilliland, B. M. (2014, April). *Enacting active shooter safety plans for postsecondary institutions.* Retrieved from http://www.pupnmag.com/media/2014/4.14/articles/0414_S&S_Creighton.pdf

Gray, R. H. (2012, August). 27 emergency notification best practices. *Campus Safety Magazine.* Retrieved from http://www.campussafetymagazine.com/article/27-emergency-notification-best-practices

Greene, H., & Greene, M. (2008, April). *What families think: Campus safety and violence.* Retrieved from http://www.universitybusiness.com/article/what-families-think-campus-safety-and-violence

Harnisch, T. L. (2008, November). *Concealed weapons on state college campuses: In pursuit of individual liberty and collective security.* Retrieved from http://www.aascu.org/WorkArea/DownloadAsset.aspx?id=4545

Hephner LaBanc, B., Krepel, T. L., Johnson, B. J., & Herrmann, L. V. (2010). Managing the whirlwind: Responding to a campus in crisis. In B. O. Hemphill & B. Hephner LaBanc (Eds.), *Enough is enough* (pp. 53–81). Sterling, VA: Stylus.

Hollingsworth, K. R., Dunkle, J. H., & Douce, L. (2009). The high-risk (disturbed and disturbing) college student. *New Directions for Student Services, 128,* 37–54. doi:10.1002/ss.340

Jablonski, M., McClellan, G., & Zdziarski, E. (Eds.). (2008). *In search of safer communities: Emerging practices for student affairs in addressing campus violence.* Washington, DC: Student Affairs Administrators in Higher Education.

Kadison, R., & DiGeronimo, T. F. (2004). *College of the overwhelmed: The campus mental health crises and what to do about it.* San Francisco, CA: Jossey-Bass.

Major Cities Chiefs. (2009, September). *Campus security guidelines: Recommended operational policies for local and campus law enforcement agencies.* Retrieved from https://majorcitieschiefs.com/pdf/news/MCC_CampusSecurity.pdf

Mankowski, E. (2013). Antecedents to gun violence: Gender and culture. In American Psychological Association (Ed.), *Gun violence: Prediction, prevention, and policy* (pp. 13–16). Washington, DC: American Psychological Association.

McCarthy, C. (2013, December). Follow best practices for campus gun policies, procedures. *Campus Safety Magazine.* Retrieved from http://www.campussecurityreport.com/Article-Detail/follow-best-practices-for-campus-gun-policies-procedures.aspx

Moore, B. L., & Carter, A. W. (2002). Creating community in a complex research university environment. In W. McDonald & associates (Eds.), *Creating campus community: In search of Ernest Boyer's legacy* (pp. 21–43). San Francisco, CA: Jossey-Bass.

National Crime Prevention Council. (2009). *Best practices for using crime prevention through environmental design in weed and seeds sites.* Retrieved from http://www.ncpc.org/resources/files/pdf/training/Best%20Practices%20in%20CPTED%20-2.pdf

Parks, K., Wilson, N. L., & Harper, R. (2010). Returning veteran with an acquired disability: Laurie. In R. Harper, N. L. Wilson, & associates (Eds.), *More than listening: A casebook for using counseling skills in student affairs work* (pp. 165–182). Washington, DC: Student Affairs Administrators in Higher Education.

Peterson, J. K., Skeem, J., Kennealy, P., Bray, B., & Zvonkovic, A. (2014). How often and how consistently do symptoms directly precede criminal behavior among offenders with mental illness? *Law and Human Behavior, 38*(5), 430–449.

Scalora, M., Simons, A., & VanSlyke, S. (2010, February). Campus safety: Assessing and managing threats. *FBI Law Enforcement Bulletin.* Retrieved from http://www.fbi.gov/stats-services/publications/law-enforcement-bulletin/february-2010/campus-safety

Schaffhauser, D. (2007, August 1). *7 practices for emergency notification.* Retrieved from http://campustechnology.com/articles/2007/08/7-best-pratices-for-emergency-notification.aspx

Scrivner, E., Tynan, W. D., & Cornell, D. (2013). Gun violence prevention at the community level. In American Psychological Association (Ed.), *Gun violence: Prediction, prevention, and policy* (pp. 23–26). Washington, DC: American Psychological Association.

Students for Concealed Carry. (n.d.). *Empty holster protest.* Retrieved from http://concealedcampus.org

Tinker, T. L., & Vaughn, E. (2012). *Risk and crisis communications: Best practices for government agencies and non-profit organizations.* Retrieved from http://www.boozallen.com/media/file/Risk-and-Crisis-Communications-Guide.PDF

U.S. Department of Education. (2007). *Lessons learned from school crises and emergencies.* Emergency Response and Crises Management Technical Assistance Center, 2(6), 1–16. Retrieved from http://www.michigan.gov/documents/safe-schools/Active_Shooter_Schools_LL_405976_7.pdf

U.S. Department of Education. (2010). *Action guide for emergency management at institutions of higher education.* Retrieved from http://rems.ed.gov/docs/REMS_ActionGuide.pdf

U.S. Department of Homeland Security. (2013). *Guide for developing high-quality emergency operations plans.* Retrieved from http://www.dhs.gov/sites/default/files/publications/REMS%20K-12%20Guide%20508_0.pdf

U.S. Department of Homeland Security. (n.d.). *Writing guide for a memorandum of understanding (MOU).* Retrieved from http://www.safecomprogram.gov/oec/mou.pdf

U.S Department of Justice. (2005). *National summit on campus public safety: Strategies for colleges and universities in a homeland security environment.* Retrieved from http://www.nccpsafety.org/assets/files/library/NationalSummitonCampus-PublicSafety.pdf

The White House. (2013, January 16). *Now is the time.* Retrieved from http://www.whitehouse.gov/sites/default/files/docs/wh_now_is_the_time_full.pdf

About the Contributors

Maggie Balistreri-Clarke is vice president for student development/dean of students at Edgewood College in Madison, Wisconsin. She also serves as chief retention officer for the college. She earned a BS from the University of Wisconsin–Stevens Point in psychology, an MS in student personnel administration and counseling and guidance at Indiana University, and a PhD in educational administration from the University of Wisconsin–Madison. She served as the NASPA Small Colleges and Universities division director and a member of NASPA Board of Directors from 2011 to 2013. She has served as a senior student affairs officer for two small colleges for over 30 years.

Ainsley Carry is vice provost for student affairs and clinical professor of educational administration at the University of Southern California. He earned a BS in food and resource economics, an MA in counselor education, and an EdD in higher education administration from the University of Florida. He also holds an MBA from Auburn University. He has served in college administration since 1998 at the University of Florida, Southern Methodist University, the University of Arkansas, Temple University, Auburn University, and currently the University of Southern California. His areas of research interest include business applications in college administration and collegiate social-innovation efforts.

Jen Day Shaw serves as associate vice president and dean of students at the University of Florida, an Association of American Universities member university of 50,000 students. In her role, she has responsibility for a 24/7 crisis response system and chairs the threat assessment team and the citywide crisis response team. She supervises the offices of student conduct and conflict resolution, new student and family programs, the disability resource center, the collegiate veterans success center, the "U Matter We Care" Program, the career resource center, and student activities and involvement. She was appointed to the VTV Family Outreach Foundation Panel of Experts, formed by the families directly impacted by the Virginia Tech tragedy. She is on the International Associations of Campus Law Enforcement Administration Accreditation Board and serves as the chair of the NASPA Campus Safety Knowledge Community. She presents widely on issues related to threat assessment. She holds a PhD from Florida State University and an MA from Miami University, Oxford, Ohio.

John H. Dunkle is executive director of counseling and psychological services (CAPS) at Northwestern University. He has been on staff at CAPS for 19 years and director for 10 years. He received his BA in psychology and his MA in experimental psychology from the State University of New York College at Cortland. He earned his PhD in counseling psychology from the University at Albany, SUNY. He is a licensed psychologist in Illinois and New York and is credentialed by the National Register of Health Service Providers in Psychology. He is a member of NASPA, the Association for University and College Counseling Center Directors, and the American Psychological Association. He has written and presented extensively on threat and risk assessment.

Rick Ferraro serves as assistant vice president for student affairs at Virginia Tech. He oversees the areas most directly associated with health and wellness, including the Schiffert Health Center, the Cook Counseling Center, recreation sports, disability services, and alcohol abuse prevention. He earned his BA in history and government from Cornell University, and he earned his MA and PhD in early modern European history from the University of Wisconsin–Madison. Having experienced, and played a significant role in a most tragic event at Virginia Tech on April 16, 2007 and having witnessed the healing and resilience brought about through the compassionate behavior of so many community members, despite the serious challenge posed by societal violence, he remains optimistic about the future.

Amy Hecht serves as the vice president for student affairs at The College of New Jersey. She earned her bachelor's degrees from Florida

State University and her master's and doctoral degrees from the University of Pennsylvania. She has served in higher education since 2001 at Alpha Chi Omega Fraternity, the University of Pennsylvania, Cabrini College, Temple University, and Auburn University. She currently holds a faculty appointment at The College of New Jersey. She also serves in leadership roles in the National Association of Student Personnel Administrators. Her areas of research interest include leadership development, organizational learning, and organizational development.

Brian O. Hemphill joined West Virginia State University as the 10th president on July 1, 2012. His energetic and visionary leadership has established a commitment to excellence, created a culture of accountability, and provided student-centered service in every interaction in order for West Virginia State University to become the most student-centered research and teaching land-grant university in West Virginia and beyond. Previously, he served as vice president for student affairs and enrollment management and associate professor at Northern Illinois University, associate vice chancellor and dean of students at the University of Arkansas–Fayetteville, associate dean of students at the University of North Carolina–Wilmington, assistant dean of students at Cornell College, and coordinator of minority recruitment and retention at Iowa State University. He earned a PhD in higher education administration from the University of Iowa, an MS in journalism and mass communication from Iowa State University, and a BA in organizational communication from St. Augustine's University. As part of his professional and scholarly work, he is a strong advocate for campus safety, following his personal experiences during the February 2008 incident at Northern Illinois University.

Steve Jacobson is the senior associate vice president at the University of the Pacific and is responsible for oversight of student activities and government, leadership programs, student life advancement and development, Greek life, community involvement programs, student life technology, educational equity programs, and crisis management. He joined Pacific in 2002 and soon thereafter began overseeing student housing, residential life, Greek life, and dining services. He received his BA from Washington State University, his MEd from Plymouth State University, and his EdD in educational administration from the University of the Pacific. From 2010 to 2014, following the leadership of Brandi Hephner LaBanc, he served as the national coordinator of Enough Is Enough, a campaign sponsored by NASPA that aims to reduce and prevent societal violence on college campuses and in their surrounding communities.

Lance Jones is the director of security and judicial review at Casper College in Casper, Wyoming. He has worked in campus law enforcement since 1991, holding positions including chief of police at 2- and 4-year public and private institutions, as well as in K–12 education and homeland security. He is a scholar and teacher of Holocaust history and has been awarded fellowships by several organizations dedicated to the study of this field. He holds an MS in occupational technology from the University of Houston and an MA in history from the University of St. Thomas.

Brandi Hephner LaBanc serves as the vice chancellor for student affairs at the University of Mississippi. She oversees departments charged with student enrollment, engagement, accountability, wellness, and inclusion. She earned a BS in accounting from the University of Akron, an MEd in higher education administration and college student personnel from Kent State University, and an EdD in adult and higher education from Northern Illinois University. As a lead campus responder during the campus shooting at Northern Illinois University in February 2008, she is motivated by her personal experience to raise awareness related to societal violence and the influence it may have on college campuses and student safety.

Sheila Lambert is the director of the wellness center at Southern New Hampshire University in Manchester, New Hampshire and oversees all health, counseling, and wellness education. She serves as a leader on the student affairs leadership team, is the cochair of the behavioral intervention team, and is chair of the Enough Is Enough committee. She has served most recently on the national Enough Is Enough advisory board and is the NASPA New Hampshire state director. Lambert has a 27-year history working in the field of mental health and substance abuse counseling and is a master's-level licensed alcohol and drug abuse counselor. She has been working in higher education for the past 12 years, specifically working with the at-risk student population. She received an undergraduate degree in health education from Plymouth State University, a master's degree in chemical dependency from LaSalle University, and a master's degree in organizational leadership from Southern New Hampshire University. She has made a longstanding effort and commitment to work with campuses around violence prevention and promotion of peace.

Jeanna Mastrodicasa is the assistant vice president for student affairs at the University of Florida where she works with the $95 million budget assessment, strategic planning, publications, and information and in the arenas of technology, and the Reitz Scholars Leadership Program. In her role at the University of Florida, she supports the work of the division of student affairs and its several departments. She is the coauthor of the 2007 book *Connecting to the Net.Generation: What Higher Education Professionals Need to Know About Today's Students*, as well as several book chapters and journal articles related to the role of technology in the life of millennials. She holds a doctoral degree in higher education administration from the University of Florida, a law degree from the University of Georgia, and a master's degree in college student personnel from the University of Tennessee. She earned her undergraduate degree in public relations from the University of Georgia.

Peter Meagher is a core faculty member at Walden University in the School of Social Work. During the past decade, he has worked and consulted with a number of higher education institutions on intervening in and preventing violence. Meagher served as director for the Campus Safety Project, an initiative to intervene in and prevent sexual assault, dating violence, and stalking. His dissertation on the use of restorative justice on the college campus won Association for Student Conduct Administrators Dissertation of the Year Award. More recently, he worked as the assistant dean of students at Gustavus Adolphus College and the associate dean of students at Reed College in Portland, Oregon.

Kerry Brian Melear is interim chair of the department of leadership and counselor education and associate professor of higher education at the University of Mississippi. His areas of expertise are college and university law, finance, and public policy. He is a member of the Author's Committee of *West's Education Law Reporter*, a member of the editorial board of the *Journal of Cases in Education*, the book review editor for the *Journal of Law & Education*, and a contributing editor to the *Higher Education Law Blog*. He has worked as a higher education policy analyst for the Florida legislature, a research associate for the Florida Postsecondary Education Commission, and an auditor for a Big Six accounting firm. He was honored to receive the University of Mississippi School of Education's Outstanding Researcher Award in 2007, 2010, and 2013 and was selected for membership on the Fulbright Specialist Roster in 2012.

Brian J. Mistler is a seasoned educator and administrator with experience both inside and outside the classroom at large public and small private institutions. He serves on the boards of the Center for Collegiate Mental Health and NASPA's *Journal of Student Affairs Research and Practice* and is a member of the Association of Threat Assessment Professionals. As associate dean of students at one of North America's preeminent private art and design colleges, he has developed a deep understanding of issues faced by senior administrators. With a PhD in psychology and postgraduate training in forensic psychology, he has gathered benchmark data for the Association for University and College Counseling Center Directors, served as an invited speaker on issues of threat assessment and campus violence prevention at the national level, and published widely on emerging social justice issues in top journals, including *LGBT Issues in Counseling*, *Transgender Studies Quarterly*, and the *Journal of Muslim Mental Health*. Proficient in risk management, compliance, and current legal trends, he has also served as Title IX coordinator for New College of Florida and on the faculty of NASPA's Higher Ed Law Certificate Program and Manatee Memorial Hospital.

Greg Nayor currently serves as the vice president of student affairs at Daemen College, and is responsible for the student life experience, including the management and supervision of the areas of student activities, residence life, counseling and health services, dining services, and campus safety. Additionally, he has served as associate faculty with Drexel University for nearly five years. Previously, he held leadership positions at the University of the Arts, Virginia Intermont

College, and Lynchburg College. An energetic and innovative leader, he has served on various committees and organizations at the state and national level. He holds a BA in history and secondary education and an MEd from the State University of New York (SUNY) College at Potsdam, as well as a PhD in higher education administration from the University of Virginia.

Scott Peska serves as the dean for students at Waubonsee Community College and has oversight of athletics, student life, student conduct, and learning assessment (testing). He earned his PhD in higher education administration with an emphasis on community college executive leadership from the University of Illinois at Urbana–Champaign. He earned both his BS in broadcast communication and his MS in communication from Illinois State University. Having led Northern Illinois University's office of support & advocacy, a unit designed to provide assistance to those individuals directly impacted by the mass shootings experienced in February 2008, he is passionate about helping educational communities enhance victim support services and move forward after violent tragic events.

Katrina A. Slone works in university relations and operations at West Virginia State University. Her work is animated by a love of syntax, grammar, and structure. Before joining the State family, she managed a small, local television station in Kentucky, where she served as graphic designer, produced local programming, wrote commercial scripts, and performed voice-over work. She is a national and state award-winning forensic speaker, with first-place rankings in informative speaking and prose interpretation. She holds a BA in English from Alice Lloyd College, where she graduated summa cum laude and was covaledictorian of her class.

Mark St. Louis holds a BA in political theory and constitutional democracy from Michigan State University, an MBA from Baker College, and a JD from Stetson University College of Law. After serving as center manager for the Center for Excellence in Higher Education Law and Policy, he accepted his current position of general counsel at New College of Florida. As general counsel, he oversees all legal and compliance issues for the college, including updating campus regulations regarding weapons on campus.

T. Ramon Stuart attended West Virginia University, where he earned undergraduate and graduate engineering degrees before obtaining his PhD in higher education administration at Ohio University. He currently serves as the associate provost and associate vice president for academic affairs at West Virginia State University. In this role, he has responsibility for several major administrative units while also playing an active part in the retention and success of West Virginia State University students.

Melanie V. Tucker is vice president for student affairs and enrollment management at Dickinson State University. A state-licensed and nationally certified professional counselor, she has earned an EdD in adult and higher education from Northern Illinois University, an EdS in counseling education from Southeast Missouri State University, an MEd in counselor education from the University of New Orleans, and a BA in applied psychology from Eastern Washington University. She is actively involved with Student Affairs Administrators in Higher Education (NASPA), having served on the NASPA Undergraduate Fellows Program Advisory Board and Disability Knowledge Community leadership team; the American College Personnel Association (ACPA), having served on the ACPA Equity and Inclusion Advisory Board and chaired the Standing Committee on Disability; and the Association for Higher Education and Disability (AHEAD), having served on the AHEAD Board of Directors. Additionally, she has volunteered as a trainer and counselor for disaster mental health relief with the Red Cross.

Sarah B. Westfall serves as vice president for student development and dean of students at Kalamazoo College. In addition to overseeing the division of student development, she leads the college's crisis response team. Much of her professional activity has focused on issues of particular relevance to small colleges, including crisis management. She earned her BA from DePauw University and her MS and PhD from Indiana University.

About the Designer

Yuma Nakada is a passionate and dynamic graphic designer and photographer who has been working internationally for more than 10 years. He is from Tokyo, Japan, but has called the United States home since 1999. He currently serves as the director of publications and design at West Virginia State University. His experiences focus on the many dynamics of higher education and nonprofit organizations, and his designs include print, illustration, brand identity, flash animation, and photography. His work may be viewed on his website (yumanakada .com).

Index

AACC. *See* American Association of Community Colleges
Abelson, Sara, 81, 94
abroad, campuses, 31
abuse, 80
academic challenges, 19–24, 39
ACE. *See* adverse childhood experiences
"ACE score," 79
ACPA–College Student Educators International, xvi–xvii
Active Minds (AM), 81, 83, 92–95
Active Shooter Response Training system, 221
ADA. *See* Americans With Disabilities Act
ad hoc members, 136
administrators, xvi–xvii, 42, 116, 190–91, 220, 222
  best practices for, 241–68
  crisis communication and mindfulness of, 177–81
  intervention readiness determined by, 104
  student development theory on gun debate and, 103–6
  tragedy and, 229–30, 235–39
adverse childhood experiences (ACE)
  category groupings of, 79
  intimate partner violence and, 79–81
  mental health issues and, 78–81
  risks of exposure to, 79–80
  study results and risk factors of, 78–79

substance abuse as most common, 79
advocacy
  concealed carry, 258
  for guns on campuses, 113–14
  for mental health, 93
African Americans, 13, 16, 18, 36–37, 166, 168, 203, 229
  hatred toward, 207
AFT. *See* American Federation of Teachers
Alaska, 63–64
Albinson, Erik, 82–83, 91
alcohol. *See* substance abuse
alert, lockdown, inform, counter, evacuate, (ALICE), 221
alerts, 251
alert system, 173
ALICE. *See* alert, lockdown, inform, counter, evacuate
alter egos, 16
Alvira, Andrea Nicole, 33
AM. *See* Active Minds
American Association of Community Colleges (AACC), 202–3
American College Health Association, 76, 84
American Federation of Teachers (AFT), 206
Americans with Disabilities Act (ADA), 126, 144, 246
  students and, 44–46
  studies and reinterpretation of, 45, 49n20
  TATs and, 135
ammunition, 64

handle problematic issues, and the need for mechanisms that allow employees and students to report problems without fear of retribution. Creating an atmosphere of transparency, accountability, and ethical behavior isn't something a leader does when a scandal strikes to protect a reputation; it's what leaders must do to reinforce their good name every day.

22883 Quicksilver Drive
Sterling, VA 20166-2102   Subscribe to our e-mail alerts: www.Styluspub.com

Also available from Stylus

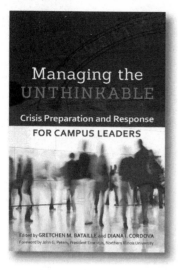

Managing the Unthinkable

Crisis Preparation and Response for Campus Leaders

Edited by Gretchen M. Bataille and Diana I. Cordova

Foreword by John G. Peters

"*Managing the Unthinkable* is absolutely a must-read for campus leadership. The insights provided by these firsthand, expert accounts of crisis management will go a long way toward helping campuses create cultures of effective, as well as immensely sensitive, responsiveness.

"The honesty in this work is breathtaking, and I applaud the authors sharing their invaluable lessons learned with such detail and clarity. It's highly readable, engrossing even. Nowhere else will you find a more comprehensive, up-to-date, and strikingly thoughtful guide to building crisis management into any campus's protocol."
—*Nancy L. Zimpher*, Chancellor, The State University of New York

Through the examples of those who have successfully managed crises, this book provides expert insights and guidance on preparedness, assigning roles and responsibilities, and planning for contingencies ahead of time so that, when there is pressure for immediate response that will be scrutinized by the media, the public, and the local constituencies, leaders can act with confidence.

The contributors emphasize the crucial importance of ethical behavior, the need for clear protocols for how all employees should

(Continues on preceding page)